FEEL GOOD

GOOD

in 15

HQ
An imprint of HarperCollins*Publishers* Ltd
1 London Bridge Street
London SE1 9GF

www.harpercollins.co.uk

HarperCollins*Publishers*
Macken House
39/40 Mayor Street Upper
Dublin 1
D01 C9W8
Ireland

10 9 8 7 6 5 4 3 2 1

First published in Great Britain by
HQ, an imprint of HarperCollins*Publishers* Ltd 2023

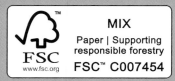

This book is produced from independently
certified FSC™ paper to ensure responsible forest
management.

For more information visit: www.harpercollins.
co.uk/green

Printed and bound by GPS in Bosnia and
Herzegovina

Publishing Director: Louise McKeever
Design Director: Laura Russell
Photographer: David Loftus
Food Stylists: Saskia Sidey and Libby Silbermann
Prop Stylist: Charlie Phillips
Designer: Nikki Ellis
Editor: Rachael Kilduff
Recipe Advisor: Saskia Sidey
Stylist: Karen Smyth
Hair and Make-up: Jo Clayton
Design Assistant: Lily Wilson
Medical Expert: Dr Mirza Marican
Senior Production Controller: Halema Begum

Thank you to Reiss and lululemon for lending us
clothing for the shoot.

When using kitchen appliances please always follow
the manufacturer's instructions.

FEEL GOOD in 15

15-MINUTE RECIPES, WORKOUTS + HEALTH HACKS

JOE WICKS

THE NO.1 BESTSELLING AUTHOR

CONTENTS

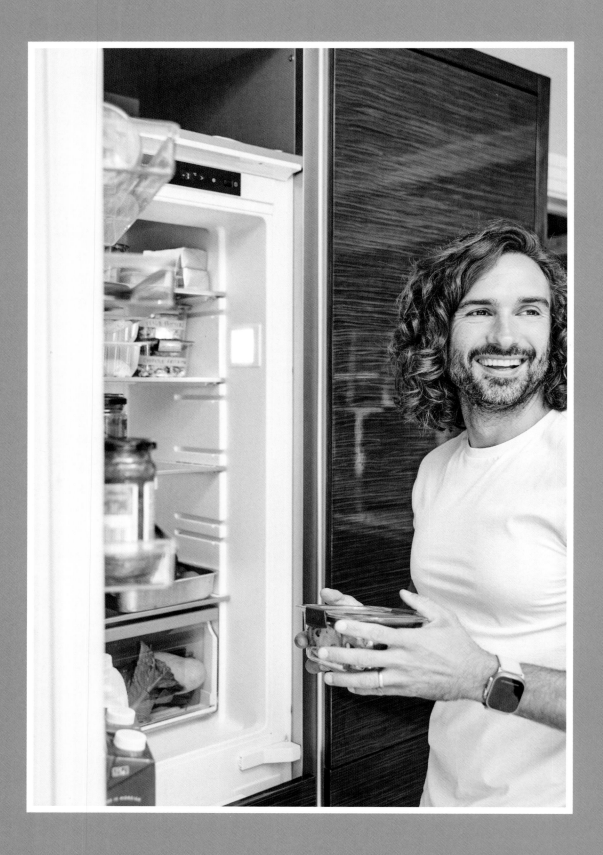

WELCOME

WOULD YOU BELIEVE ME IF I SAID YOU COULD START TO CHANGE YOUR LIFE TODAY WITH JUST 15 MINUTES?

It sounds a bit ambitious, I know, but believe me because I live by a principle I like to call 'small daily wins' and it has helped me in so many ways. Small daily wins mean finding a short window of time every day to do one or a few positive things to make you feel good. This could be anything from cooking a quick, healthy recipe to moving your body for 15 minutes or simply getting to bed earlier. Fifteen minutes is not a long time and in isolation it will not transform your mind or body, but all the small daily wins start to add up and compound over weeks, months and eventually years. Small actions can create big changes in your life. I really do believe that, and I've seen the impact this mindset can have on people, especially those who lead busy, stressful lives. Stress is one of the biggest factors in determining someone's overall health and well-being, so if we can reduce stress and make daily life feel a bit easier, these new daily habits can stick.

This book contains 60 delicious 15-minute meals that I think you will love, but it's also so much more than just a cookbook. This is a guide to help you get fitter, healthier and ultimately happier. It's full of my best tips, ideas and strategies to create real change in your life and start to feel good. I've worked with almost 1 million people on The Body Coach app over the past 10 years and I've taken everything I have learned and packed it into the chapters of this book.

The biggest and most impactful lesson I have learned from all my years as a health and fitness coach is the importance of time. Time is short, time is precious and time is everything when it comes to living a happy, healthy life. 'I don't have time to cook.' 'I haven't got enough time to fit in exercise.' 'I wish I had more time to look after myself.' These are the most common things I hear people say, but I always try to help them believe that they can find time. This book is all about giving you back time and finding practical, realistic ways of utilising 15 minutes to do something impactful. You'll be amazed at what can actually be achieved in 15 minutes. I've included healthy recipes, bodyweight HIIT routines and dumbbell strength sessions, as well as advice and techniques around sleep, mindfulness, gratitude, cold-water therapy and some fun activities to try with your family.

I want this book to help you not only to reconnect with yourself and your own mental and physical health, but hopefully to reconnect with friends and family too, in a way that brings everyone a little bit more joy. These are values and principles I believe are essential to a happy life. Remember, not every day will be perfect and there are always going to be challenges that slow you down, but with the right mindset you can find 15 minutes each day to take on life's challenges – and win.

Thank you so much for giving this book a go. I hope it helps you find a little bit more energy and happiness in your life. Good luck!

Much love,

Joe

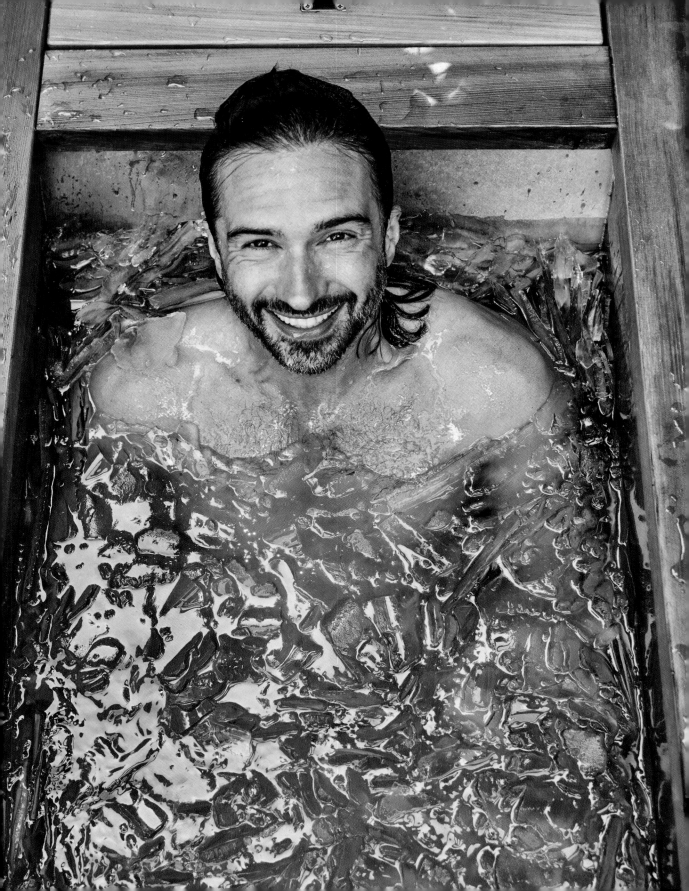

Fast food is what I'm known for, but I definitely do not mean the takeaway stuff that is pre-made and you buy on the way home. Fast food to me is the healthy recipes you whip up in your kitchen at home.

I built my whole online community with the 'Lean in 15' concept, which was all about making delicious and healthy recipes in under 15 minutes. I've gone off and done longer meals in the past and even had a crack with a 30-minute recipe book, but the truth is, people always respond best to my shorter recipes. So here I am back with what I believe are my best recipes yet. I know I say that every time, lol, but I really do mean it this time. Every single one of these recipes I've created, tried and tested and continue to make on a regular basis for Rosie, the kids and me. So have a browse through, maybe favourite the best ones with a Post-It note and get cooking. Be adventurous and try something new. After all, variety is the spice of life, isn't it?

15-MINUTE MEALS

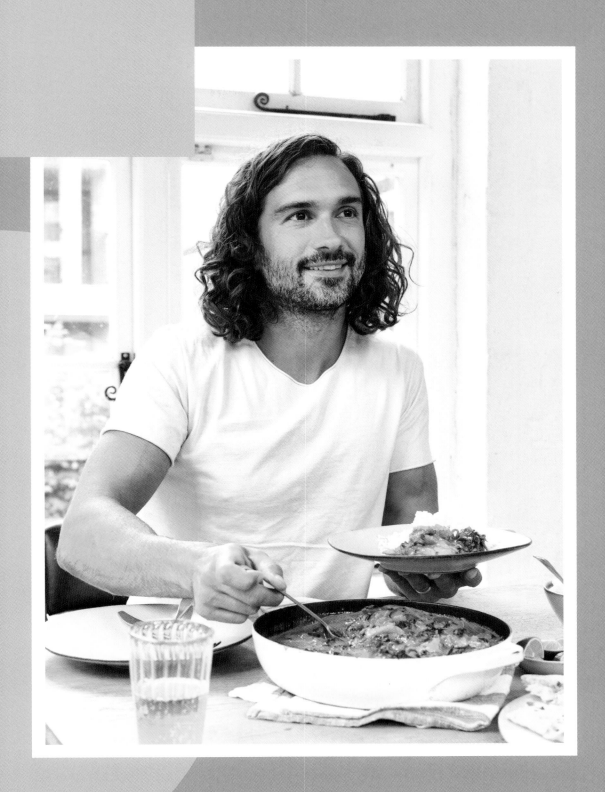

PLANNING WILL MAKE YOUR LIFE EASIER

Life has a way of getting in the way and we can often end up relying on convenience, processed and fast foods on the go to fuel ourselves. But by sitting down for 15 minutes on a weekend and planning out your week ahead, taking into account the foods you would like to eat and the ingredients you need, you are setting yourself up for future success. You can then do your weekly shop in store or online knowing you are filling your basket with all the good stuff you need to fuel your body.

Personally, I like to batch cook certain meals, so I always make sure I have my store-cupboard essentials and all the ingredients I need for my favourite quick and healthy breakfasts, lunches and dinners. Speed is everything, I think, and it's so important when it comes to sticking to a healthy diet. Plan meals like the ones in this book which are ready in under 15 minutes, and where possible, double up recipes and batch cook so you have some leftovers for the following day. It's very hard to fall off track if every day you head off to work with your own prepared lunch or you return home with a meal in the fridge just ready to be reheated.

Keeping organised will change your life and will help you feel good and lose weight because you are in control of what you are eating. It can feel stressful at first, but the more you plan and begin to get in the habit of meal prepping, the easier it becomes. Without a doubt, you will get faster at planning and cooking your favourite meals. Another bonus is the cost savings, as you will save money on your weekly food spend if you have taken the time to plan your meals for the week (see pages 14–15).

WHEN YOU BUY IN BULK AND COOK MORE AT HOME, YOU WILL SAVE MONEY ON YOUR WEEKLY FOOD SPEND. A WIN-WIN!

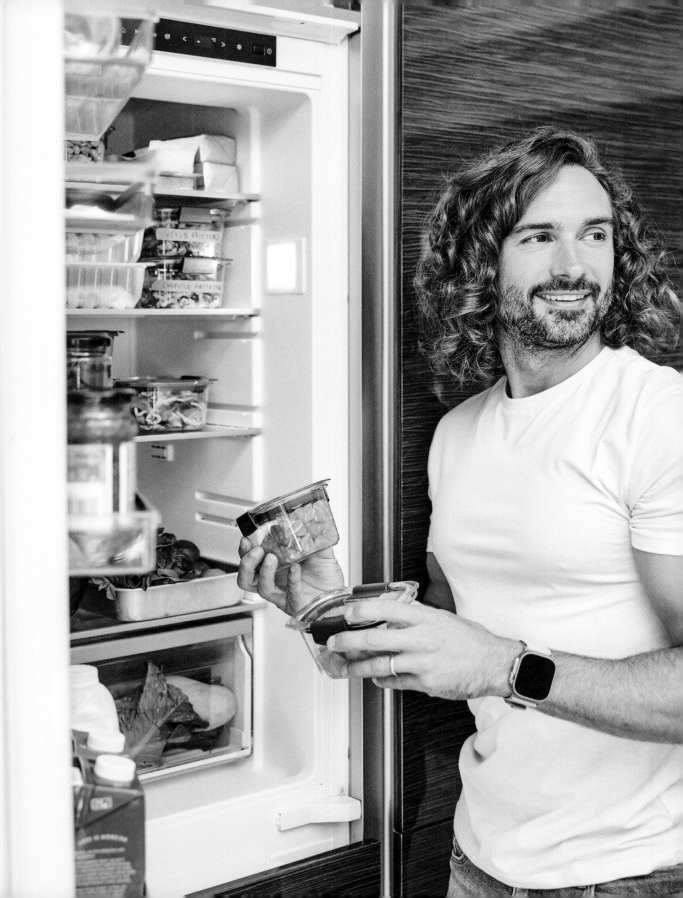

PREPPING LIKE A BOSS

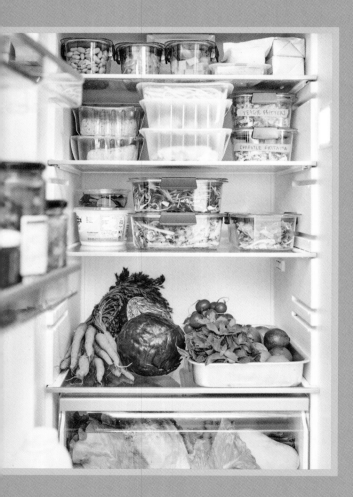

I really believe speed is everything when it comes to eating healthy – make it fast and you can keep it healthy and stay on track to achieve your goals. The recipes in this book reflect that because I've designed them to be simple, quick and stress-free, so you can enjoy the foods you love and that are good for you without too much effort.

If you follow me on social media or use The Body Coach app, you'll have heard me talk about 'Prepping Like a Boss'. While I do believe that a balanced and flexible approach to eating is best for long-term success in creating a sustainable and enjoyable diet, it's really helpful to do a bit of planning, too. Just making a few decisions on recipes and drawing up a plan for your daily meals once a week can save you a lot of time and effort on a day-to-day basis. Do this and you'll know exactly what you need to buy and you'll have everything on hand and ready to cook – you will be amazed at how much you can achieve in 15 minutes if you get organised.

TIP ←

When you are planning each week, give yourself a free flexible lazy day on which you can pull something from the freezer, eat up leftovers or chuck a load of odds and ends into a pan to avoid food waste.

HOW TO DO IT

Block out 15 minutes once a week when you sit down and do your planning for all of your meals for the week. Think about when you will need lunches for work and days you will be out in the evening. This might seem like an effort at first, but as you get more familiar with it, it will quickly become part of your weekly routine. Here are a few tips for success:

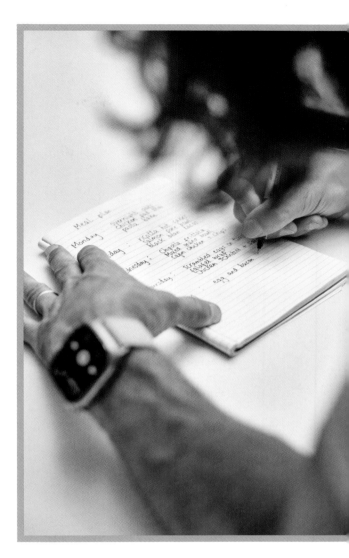

1 Draw on a piece of paper each day of the week, or use the in-app planner on The Body Coach app. Write down 3 meals and 2 snacks every day using any of my recipes from my books or online. Try to choose recipes that really appeal to you and other people in your household, if you are cooking for more than one – if it's food you will enjoy, you are more likely to cook it and stick to the plan. Don't forget to include any leftovers or think about making a little bit more – this can give you great lunch options (see page 21).

2 If you can fit in a batch-cooking session once a week to get ahead, this will make dinner on a busy night really simple, as you can pull out a home-cooked meal from the fridge or freezer and just heat it up. It also means less waste, because if you change your plans one day and need to shuffle your meals around, it can stay in the freezer for another day (see page 23).

3 Once you've got your plan, check your cupboards, fridge and freezer and make a list of the ingredients you need for your meals and snacks for the week (see pages 18–19), then place your online order or hit the shops. Doing a big shop is a really good way to stick to your food goals – deciding exactly what you need to buy helps you avoid those 'top-up' trips when you can end up picking up unhealthy ready meals, treats or even fast food on the go. It also saves both time and money, as it avoids food being left uneaten and wasted at the end of the week.

15 STORE-CUPBOARD HEROES THAT EVERY HOME NEEDS

Alright, listen up, folks! If you're tired of spending hours in the kitchen, slaving away over a hot stove, then this book is about to change your life. We all need a few tricks up our sleeves to help us save time without compromising on flavour or quality. In our busy lives, finding the time to prepare delicious and nutritious meals can often feel like an impossible task. The following versatile ingredients are the backbone of the recipes that follow in this book. These store-cupboard heroes will become your trusty companions, helping you to make mouthwatering dishes that can be prepared in just 15 minutes – taking the stress out of your busy day and meaning making good choices is much easier.

CHILLI JAM

A little jar of this is the perfect balance of sweet and spicy. Use it to glaze meats, as a dipping sauce, or to spice up your sandwiches.

CHIPOTLE

This smoky little devil paste is a spicy and rich Mexican ingredient that adds incredible depth and complexity to recipes. It's great mixed into marinades and dressings, and is perfect for quick fajitas, burritos and stews.

CURRY PASTE

If you've got a jar of curry paste in the cupboard, you're never going to skimp on flavour. Bursting with fragrant spices, curry paste instantly adds depth and complexity to your dishes with hardly any effort – I always keep a mild curry paste on hand, but I also love a Thai green curry paste.

HARISSA PASTE

Infuse your dishes with a fiery kick using harissa paste. This North African spice blend adds a vibrant and aromatic flavour to your recipes. From marinades to dips, harissa paste injects a perfectly balanced bit of heat to any dish.

KIMCHI

This tangy, fermented cabbage is spicy, full of umami flavours and packed with probiotics to support your gut. I love adding it to stir-fries, rice bowls or even grilled cheese toasties for a zesty kick and gut health boost.

LIME PICKLE

This Indian condiment delivers a burst of citrusy goodness to your dishes. Enjoy it as a dip, spread it on sandwiches, or use it to elevate your curries and rice dishes.

MICROWAVE RICE + GRAIN POUCHES

These time-saving marvels provide perfectly cooked and fluffy grains in minutes. Whether you're in the mood for quinoa, rice or other wholegrains, these pouches ensure you have a nutritious and versatile base for your meals in no time.

MISO PASTE

Discover the umami-rich depths of miso paste. This traditional Japanese ingredient adds a complex and savoury flavour to a wide range of recipes. From soups and broths to dressings and glazes – and even desserts – miso paste allows you to create delicious and comforting meals with ease.

PEANUT BUTTER

We go through peanut butter in this house by the bucket-load. Creamy and nutty goodness that adds richness and depth, whether you're blending it into smoothies, using it as the base for a sauce or satay; it's always got a place in my kitchen.

PERI-PERI SAUCE

We all know and love a bit of peri-peri – this hot sauce packs a punch. Use it to marinate meats, add a kick to your grilled dishes or spice up your burgers and sandwiches.

PESTO

There's so much more to pesto than pasta. Traditionally made with basil, garlic, nuts and cheese, it adds a burst of freshness to any recipe. I like to buy pesto that you find in the fridge at the supermarket rather than a jar, but both will work here.

PICKLED JALAPENOS

These zesty pickled chillies add a punch of heat and tang – perfect for Mexican-inspired dishes, sandwiches and even pizzas. We've used them in a burger sauce in this book because I can't get enough of the spice.

SUN-DRIED TOMATOES

Add a burst of intense flavour to your dishes with sun-dried tomatoes. They're concentrated in sweetness and are so good in salads, used in pasta sauces, or incorporated into bread and dips. They're a little taste of sunshine.

TAHINI

Tahini is so creamy and nutty – the sesame-seed paste is traditionally used in Middle Eastern cuisine but it can also be fabulous with flavours like soy and rice vinegar for an Asian twist. It's super-smooth and rich. I love drizzling a bit over yoghurt and berries for a quick breakfast.

TAMARIND SAUCE

This is bold, sweet, tangy and super-versatile. It's epic in marinades, dressings and dipping sauces, and you'll find the taste quite familiar because it's the base of HP Sauce!

WHAT TO BUY

Eating well – and getting food on the table quickly – feels good, and is made much easier by having the right foods (and none of the wrong foods). Keeping your kitchen well-stocked is a key part of prepping, so when you do your weekly meal planning, have a quick check in your cupboards, fridge and freezer to see what you need to buy and what might need using up.

This cupboard list includes items that feature in these recipes, but most of them are also my favourite standby ingredients that I have to hand at all times, as I use them over and over again. Some are a little more unusual and possibly a bit more expensive to buy, so they aren't in every recipe. You don't need them all. The fridge, freezer and fresh food lists are specific to the recipes in this book.

FREEZER

berries (all kinds: blueberries, strawberries, raspberries)
mixed vegetables
peas
raw king prawns
vanilla ice cream

FRESH

apples
asparagus
aubergines
avocados
bananas
blueberries
bread (bagels, burger buns, ciabatta, crumpets, flatbreads, naan/chapatis, sliced loaf, sourdough)
broccoli
Brussels sprouts
butternut squash
cabbages (red, Savoy)
carrots
chillies
chives
citrus fruit (grapefruit, lemons, limes, oranges)

courgettes
cucumber
edamame beans
fresh ginger
garlic
gnocchi
green beans
herbs (basil, coriander, dill, mint, oregano, parsley, rosemary, tarragon, thyme)
kimchi
kiwis
leeks
lemongrass
mango
mushrooms
onions (white, red, shallots)
pak choi
peaches

peppers
plums
pomegranates
potatoes (baby, baking)
radishes
raspberries
salad (lamb's lettuce, Little Gem, mixed leaves, rocket, romaine, watercress)
spinach or kale
spring onions
strawberries
sugar snap peas
sweet potatoes
tomatoes (cherry, salad)
tortilla wraps

CUPBOARD

apricot jam
baking powder
bicarbonate of soda
black treacle
chilli jam
chipotle paste
coconut milk
cornflour
corn tacos
couscous
curry paste
dark chocolate
dates
digestives
dried cranberries
dried herbs and spices
   (cayenne pepper, chilli
   flakes, cinnamon,
   coriander, cumin, fajita
   seasoning, garam masala,
   ginger, mixed spice,
   oregano, paprika, turmeric)
eggs
flour (gram, plain, self-raising)
ginger nut biscuits
harissa
honey
hot sauce
jar of beetroot in vinegar
jar of capers
jar of pickled jalapenos
jar of roasted red peppers
jar of stem ginger in syrup
jar of sun-dried tomatoes
ketchup/tomato sauce/
   passata
lemon curd
lime pickle
mango chutney
maple syrup
marmalade
Marmite
marshmallows
mayonnaise
meringue kisses/nests

microwave grain sachets
   (quinoa, puy lentils)
microwave rice sachets
   (brown, long-grain, risotto
   and sticky or jasmine)
miso paste
mustard (Dijon, yellow)
'nduja paste
nuts (flaked almonds,
   hazelnuts, pecans, pine
   nuts, pistachios, salted
   peanuts)
oils and oil spray (chilli, light
   and extra-virgin olive,
   sesame, vegetable)
oyster sauce
panko breadcrumbs
pasta (orzo, penne, spaghetti
   or bucatini)
peanut butter
peri-peri sauce
pesto
porridge oats
quick-cook polenta
ras el hanout
sea salt and black pepper
seeds (chia, nigella, pumpkin,
   sesame, sunflower)
soy sauce
stock cubes (beef, chicken,
   vegetable)
sugar (caster, demerara)
tahini
tamarind sauce
tin of artichoke hearts
tin of dulce de leche
tin of Kalamata olives
tins or pouches of cooked
   pulses (black beans, butter
   beans, cannellini beans,
   chickpeas, kidney, lentils)
tins of tomatoes/sweetcorn
vanilla extract
vinegar (apple cider, balsamic,
   red/white wine, sesame)

FRIDGE

bacon
beef (mince, steaks)
butter
cheese (Cheddar, cream,
   feta, halloumi, Manchego,
   mozzarella, Parmesan,
   ricotta)
chicken (breasts, thighs)
chorizo
cod
cottage cheese
double cream
falafels
Greek yoghurt
lamb (mince)
milk (of choice)
natural yoghurt
pancetta cubes
Parma ham
pork belly strips
ready-to-roll pastry (filo, puff)
salmon (fresh, smoked)
sausages
soured cream
tomato purée concentrate

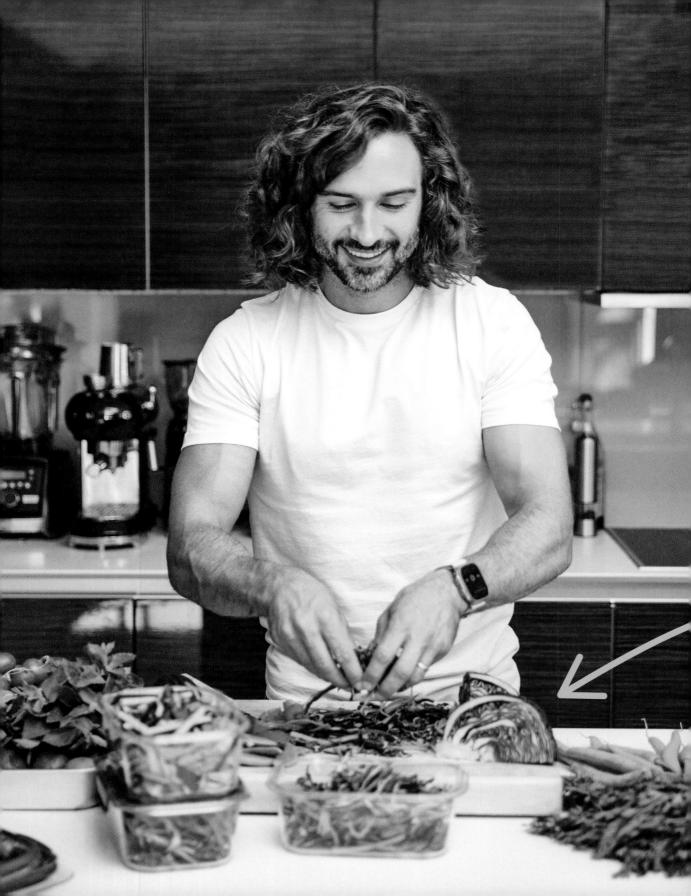

BATCH IT UP NOW

We all have those days when we don't feel good – we get in late after work and feel exhausted and overwhelmed, and even having 15 minutes to make a healthy dinner feels too much. Instead, save yourself a little time, block out a couple of hours on a Sunday afternoon and smash out some food to keep in your freezer for those busy nights. You will thank yourself later.

PRE-COOKED MEALS WILL LAST UP TO 3–4 DAYS IN THE FRIDGE AND UP TO 1 MONTH IN THE FREEZER.

Batch cooking is a brilliant way of staying on track; with a little bit of planning you can prep some grab-and-go breakfasts, packed lunches and speedy dinners for as many days as you like – for example, in 15 minutes you could prep 3 days' worth of overnight oats for breakfast, or 3 days' worth of orzo pasta for lunch. Doing this once a week is really helpful and will set you up for a good few days, but you can have another go mid-week if you like to make life really easy.

So get ahead and either batch cook some delicious food that you can stick in the freezer or enjoy over the next few days, or if you don't fancy cooking or don't have time for that, simply preparing and chopping fresh ingredients for your chosen recipes for the next day can really help save precious time later.

Batch cooking is really easy: you just double or triple the quantities in a recipe to serve as many people as you'd like, cook away in one go, then portion up and store. This is where a boss prepper knows the value of having loads of Tupperware or similar freezerproof containers knocking about. If you don't have any, invest in about eight large-ish containers for full meals, and a few smaller ones for snacks and lunchboxes.

It's worth getting a few labels for your boxes, too, because if you become a batch-cooking pro you'll need to know what is in each container as you pull them out of the freezer!

DON'T WASTE YOUR FOOD

We all want to cut down on the amount of food that we chuck away, so how can you make sure you're only buying what you need? Yep, you guessed it, prepping is key to keeping food waste to a minimum. Here are a few tips to help you use what you have:

1 Stick to the plan: when you plan your weekly meals you are also creating a shopping list, so stick to it and try to avoid buying any extras (see page 27).

2 Eat in order: always rotate your ingredients when you buy new ones, moving those with the oldest sell-by/use-by dates to the front so that you use them first before they expire.

3 Cook only what you know you will eat – stick to your portion sizes, or if you do cook too much and have leftovers, let them cool completely if cooked, then cover and store them in the fridge or freezer to eat later, or eat them for lunch the next day. Leftovers can be stored in the fridge for a maximum of 4 days.

4 Storing in the fridge or freezer: knowing what you can freeze and what is best kept in the fridge will help you avoid wasting food, as well as the time you've taken to prep it. As a general rule, curries, sauces and casseroles are great for freezing, and you'll find many recipes in this book that you can make in large batches and freeze. To freeze, make sure the food has cooled completely in a sealed freezerproof container (don't forget to label it!) before placing it in the freezer. To eat, defrost overnight in the fridge, or in the microwave for a speedy supper. Once defrosted, cook for 5–10 minutes or until piping hot throughout.

TIP:

Do your bit for the planet and keep your food costs down by buying 'imperfect' veg and fruit. Each year around the world about 1.3 billion tonnes of food is rejected by supermarkets for not meeting their aesthetic standards and is thrown out – that's almost 40% of crops harvested. But now you can rescue these ingredients, which are offered for sale in supermarkets and online box schemes for less than the price of the perfect varieties. So do your bit and buy ugly!

WHEN FROZEN IS BETTER THAN FRESH

We know that fruit and veggies should form the backbone of a healthy and nutritious diet, and when we think about including these ingredients it's often the fresh version we reach for. However, leave these in the fridge or the fruit bowl for too long and they will start to go past their best.

Frozen fruit and veg, on the other hand, can be stored for between 6 and 10 months without deteriorating, and it is as healthy as, if not healthier than, fresh, because it is packaged and frozen very quickly after being picked at peak ripeness. This is when it is at its most nutritious, having had very little time for its nutrients to degrade, whereas fresh fruit and veg is picked before it becomes ripe, when it has not yet developed a full range of nutrients. (It's worth noting that buying ready chopped fresh fruit and veg in those bags or tubs may be a time saver in the kitchen but they might also be a less nutritious option, as some of the nutrients – such as vitamins A, C and E – can be lost once the ingredients are sliced and the flesh is exposed to oxygen.)

Frozen fruit and veg is really handy to keep in the freezer for those days when you don't have fresh veg or you don't have time to prep and chop vegetables for cooking – you can simply defrost or tip the ingredients out of the packet straight into the recipe as part of your five a day. You can buy packs of your favourite veg individually or a mixed veg selection for a bit of variety and colour – these are perfect for soups, curries, stews, stir-fries and rice dishes.

When it comes to fruit, frozen blueberries, strawberries, raspberries, cherries and chunks of mango or peaches allow you to enjoy a taste of summer all year round, and you won't have to rush to eat them before they lose their flavour and freshness. One disadvantage to frozen fruit, however, is that their texture is altered during freezing, so they do go a bit mushy. They are best used in recipes where that doesn't matter, such as blended into smoothies, cooked into crumbles, puréed into a compote for topping yoghurt or porridge, or dolloped onto pancakes.

Another great advantage of frozen fruit and veg is that they are often considerably cheaper than fresh, so along with being far less wasteful, what's not to love about these little packets of goodness?

FILL YOUR FREEZER WITH PLENTY OF FROZEN VEG

KEEPING YOUR GUT HAPPY

Gut health is important for a variety of reasons, ranging from its impact on digestion to its influence on overall wellbeing and your mental health. Diet plays a huge role in your gut health and science now shows the effects good food really does have on our mood.

DIGESTION AND NUTRIENT ABSORPTION:

A healthy gut is essential for proper digestion and absorption of nutrients from the food you eat. The gut is responsible for breaking down food into smaller particles and absorbing nutrients, including vitamins and minerals, that are necessary for overall health and functioning.

IMMUNE SYSTEM SUPPORT:

A significant portion of the immune system is located in the gut, where it helps to protect the body. A balanced and diverse community of good bacteria in the gut helps to support immune function and prevent the growth of harmful bacteria.

MOOD AND MENTAL HEALTH:

There's a strong connection between the gut and the brain. The gut produces the majority of our bodies' serotonin, a chemical that can influence mood and mental health.

WEIGHT MANAGEMENT:

The gut microbiome plays a role in regulating metabolism and energy balance, and imbalances have been linked to obesity and metabolic disorders.

TOP TIPS FOR A HAPPY GUT

To maintain good gut health, it's important to focus on a balanced and diverse diet that is rich in fibre, prebiotics (which support the growth of beneficial bacteria) and probiotics (live bacteria that are beneficial for gut health). Additionally, managing stress, staying hydrated, getting regular exercise and avoiding excessive use of antibiotics can also contribute to a healthier gut.

- Try to eat many kinds of plants. If you had carrots and parsnips last night, have courgette tonight. The more different kinds of plants you eat, the more diverse your gut microbes.

- 'Plants' doesn't just mean fruit and vegetables. There are six different plant groups: vegetables, fruits, wholegrains, legumes (beans and pulses), nuts and seeds, and herbs and spices. The more you eat from across these groups, the better.

- Focus on eating more good stuff, as opposed to cutting out bad stuff. Research has shown that adding 'good stuff' to your diet has a much greater effect on your gut health than just cutting out 'bad stuff'. Your focus should be: 'What can I add?' not 'What can I take away?'

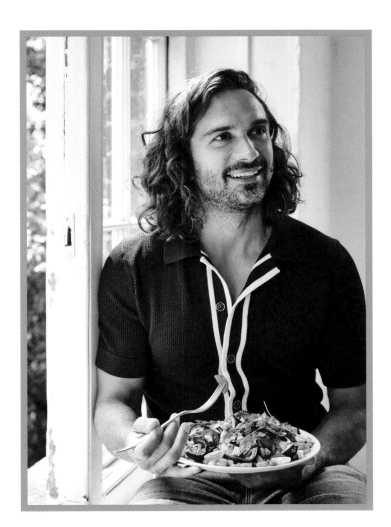

FOCUS ON EATING MORE FOODS THAT ARE GOOD FOR YOU, AS OPPOSED TO FOCUSING ON CUTTING OUT ANY BAD STUFF.

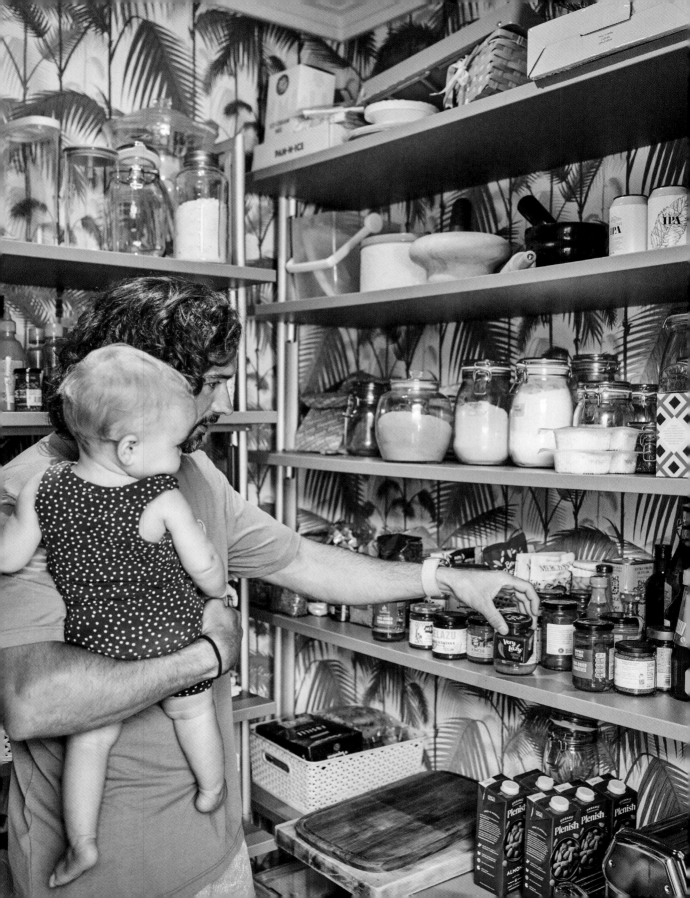

MANAGING YOUR MUNCHIES

I have good discipline with my exercise and find it very easy to be consistent with it, but when it comes to food, I find it much harder. I think lots of people struggle with food because temptation is around us all day long. When we are stressed, tired or feeling emotional, our natural response is often turning to food to make us feel better.

CHOOSE FEEL-GOOD FOOD

I'm an all-or-nothing kind of guy, so when I start eating a packet of biscuits or a bar of chocolate, I will finish the lot. I admire and respect people who can take one square of chocolate and put the rest of the bar back in the fridge, but that's just not me and I don't think it ever will be. I don't have any guilt around having a binge on chocolate or smashing a whole tub of ice cream at all, but I do feel the negative effects on my body. What I used to think of as a treat to myself, I've come to realise really isn't, and I've started to acknowledge this. Certain foods can make me feel bloated, sluggish and/or lethargic and it often affects my mood. So, I try to avoid doing this often because I want to feel good and I want to feel energised.

REMOVE THE TEMPTATION!

The only strategy which works for me is removing the temptations from the fridge and cupboards at home. If the foods I crave and binge on are not there, then I'm far more likely to stay on track with my goals of healthy eating. I'm not going to lie, I still love a treat when I'm out, and some days I'll pop round to the shop on a choccy run after a stressful day, but the daily snacking and grazing stops when it's not in my reach every day.

Next time you are doing your food shopping, think about what's going in the basket and start to reduce the foods which are your biggest temptations and those triggers for emotional eating. This simple step can really help with your willpower and discipline around food and help you to achieve your goals, especially if your goal is to lose weight.

BREAKFAST

Starting your day with breakfast as soon as you wake up isn't essential, but if you are going to do it let's get it right. You may be someone like myself who likes to train on an empty stomach and then refuels afterwards. Or you could be someone who feels more energised eating a quick breakfast before you leave the house. Don't worry, I've got you covered in this chapter with 15 of my best and most popular quick and nutritious breakfasts.

If you are someone who always feels like breakfast is a rush, then I'm confident these recipes can help you. Some can be made in a few minutes while others can be batch cooked and prepped the night before. My aim with everything is to remove stress and keep things simple so you can avoid the sugary cereals, processed breakfast bars, energy drinks or coffee that always lead to a sugar crash.

The recipes will make you feel good and fuel your body and mind. They will energise you and improve your focus and productivity so you can go on to have an awesome day.

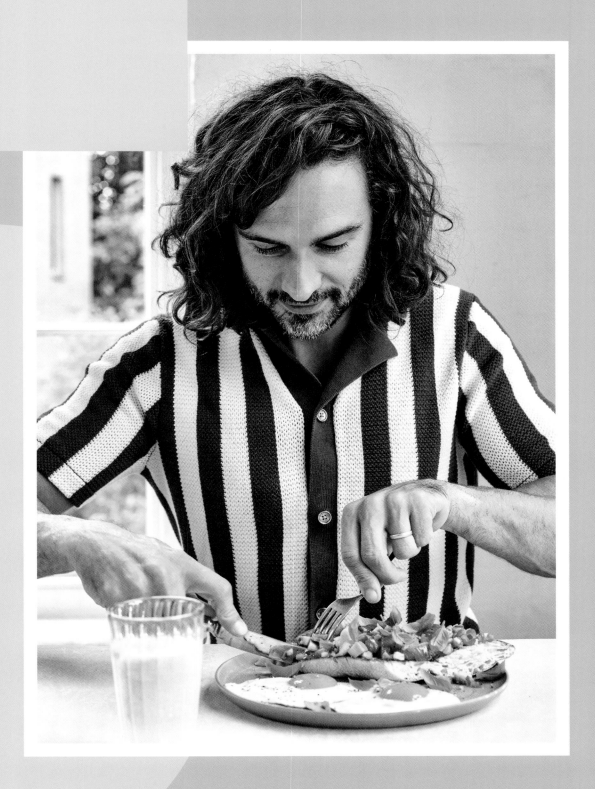

GREEK SCRAMBLE

By the beard of Zeus! Bored of plain old scrambled eggs on toast for breakfast? Spice things up with this delicious, Greek salad-inspired version: softly scrambled eggs with all the fresh, zingy salad ingredients we know and love. This is a dreamy combo full of goodness. Perfect fuel to start the day.

SERVES 2

¼ red onion, thinly sliced
4 eggs
2 tbsp milk
1 tbsp olive oil, plus extra
   to drizzle
2 slices of sourdough
100g (3½oz) cherry
   tomatoes, halved
60g (2½oz) Kalamata
   olives, stoned
¼ cucumber, sliced
40g (1½oz) feta, crumbled
handful of fresh oregano
   sprigs
salt and freshly ground
   black pepper

1 Place the sliced red onion into a small bowl and cover with cold water – this takes away the intense raw flavour.

2 In a small bowl, crack in the eggs and pour in the milk and whisk well with a fork to combine. Season generously.

3 Add 1 tablespoon of oil to a non-stick frying pan and pour in the egg mixture. Cook over a low heat, stirring regularly with a silicone spatula and scraping up the egg from the bottom and edges until you can see no more runny egg. Turn off the heat and set aside.

4 Pop the sourdough in the toaster for 2 minutes.

5 Drain the onion and arrange over the other chopped vegetables and the feta on a plate. Serve with the toasted sourdough and scrambled eggs and sprinkle the oregano sprigs over the whole lot.

TIP/SWAP

If you can't find fresh oregano, try adding a pinch of dried oregano to the eggs before you scramble them.

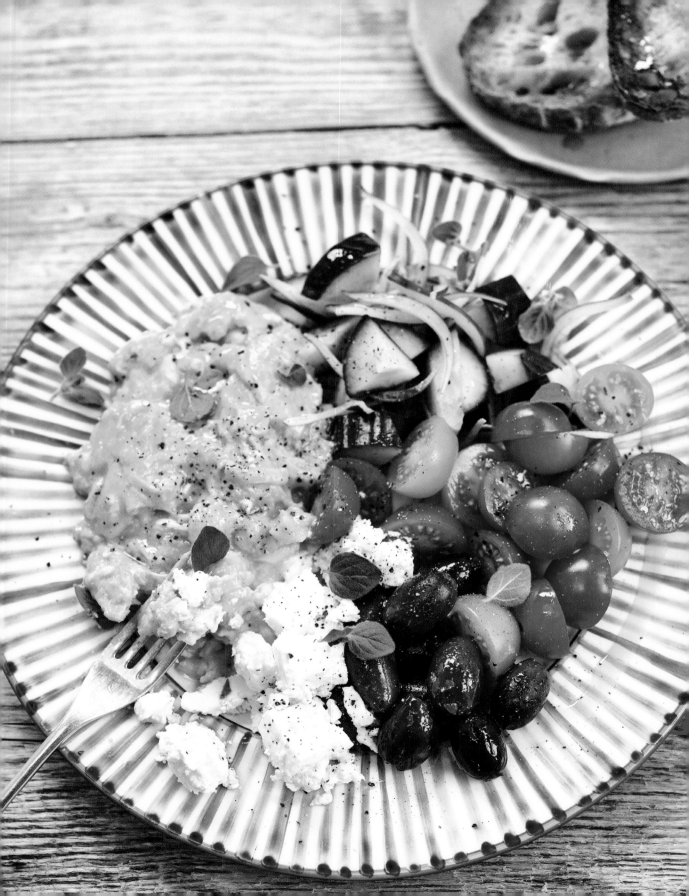

OATY PEANUT SMOOTHIE

I'm a self-confessed peanut butter nutter. I can't get enough of the stuff and my kids love it too. This smoothie can be whizzed up in no time, and I always have these ingredients knocking around. Super-filling, it's the perfect way to start your day, especially if you are in a hurry to get out the door.

SERVES 1

1 large banana
2 dates, stoned
30g (1oz) porridge oats
1½ tbsp peanut butter
  (smooth or chunky)
160ml (5½fl oz) oat milk

1 Peel the banana and add to the jug of a blender, reserving a few slices for garnish, if you like.

2 Add the dates, oats, peanut butter and oat milk.

3 Blitz until smooth, then pour into a large glass and top with banana slices, if you like.

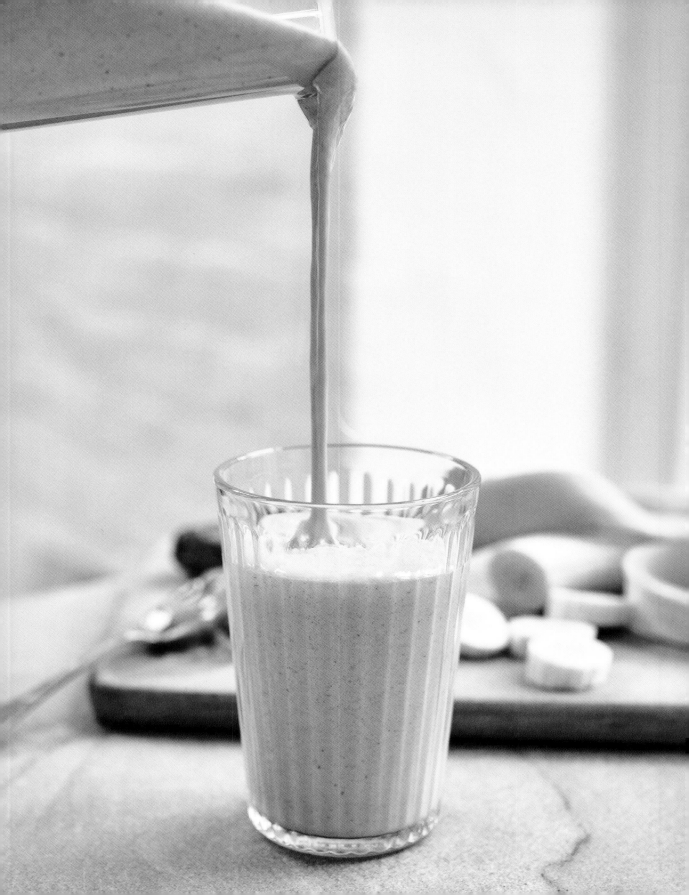

RICOTTA HOT CAKES

V

These little fluffy pancakes are as soft as clouds and absolutely perfect for the whole family to enjoy. This makes a few too many pancakes for two people, but I always hate having half a tub of ricotta left in the fridge, so follow the tip below to save the leftovers for the next day.

MAKES 8 PANCAKES

250g (9oz) ricotta
3 eggs
200ml (7fl oz) whole milk
½ tsp vanilla extract
1 tsp white wine vinegar
3 tsp baking powder
200g (7oz) plain flour
1 tbsp butter, for frying

To serve
4 tbsp thick Greek yoghurt
1–2 apples, grated
a drizzle of honey

1 In a bowl, whisk together the ricotta, eggs, milk, vanilla extract and vinegar until smooth-ish – it's OK if there are some lumps of ricotta.

2 Add the baking powder and flour and stir to combine until no dry bits of flour remain.

3 Heat a frying pan and add half of the butter. Add 2–3 tablespoons of batter to the pan for each pancake. Fry the pancakes over a medium heat for 1–2 minutes on each side until puffy, golden and risen. You'll likely have to do this in two batches, using the remaining butter to re-grease the pan.

4 Serve while hot with a dollop of Greek yoghurt, some grated apple and a drizzle of honey.

TIP/SWAP

If you can't finish all the pancakes, they freeze well and can be defrosted and warmed through in the toaster or microwave for a speedy breakfast fix.

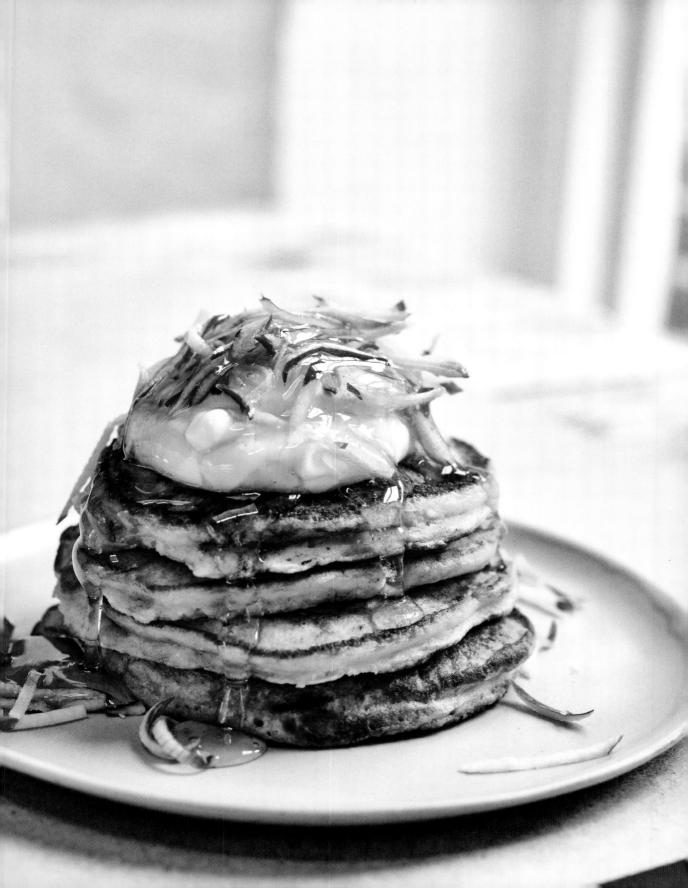

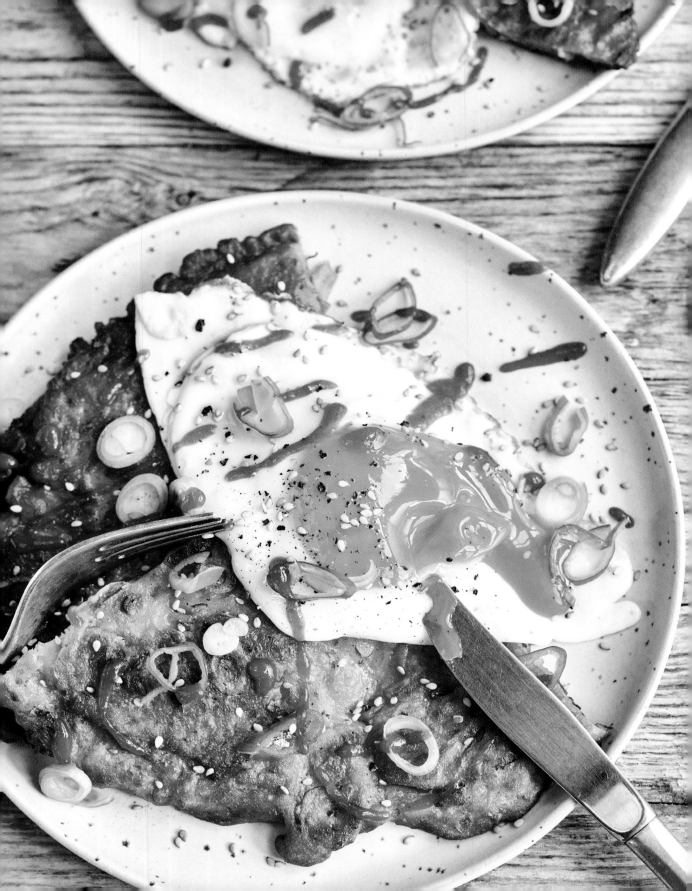

KIMCHI PANCAKES

Feeling a bit windy? Give this gut-friendly recipe a go to help settle things down. Kimchi is a spicy fermented cabbage that has lots of good bacteria, making it great for your gut. It's really tangy with a spicy kick and packs in a lot of flavour. Don't knock it until you've tried it.

SERVES 2

100g (3½oz) plain flour
3 eggs
1 tbsp soy sauce
60ml (2½fl oz) water
200g (7oz) kimchi, roughly chopped
2 spring onions, finely sliced
2 tbsp vegetable oil
1 tbsp sesame seeds (I like to buy pre-toasted)
hot sauce, to serve (optional)

1 Whisk the flour, 1 of the eggs, the soy sauce and water in a medium bowl. Stir through the kimchi and most of the spring onions, reserving a handful for garnish.

2 Heat the oil in a medium non-stick frying pan. When the oil shimmers, pour in the batter, using the back of a wooden spoon to smooth it out to the edges. Cook for 2–3 minutes on each side until golden. A little trick to flip the pancake to cook the other side is to place a large plate on top of the pan, using oven gloves, and flip the whole thing over, then slide the pancake back into the pan from the plate, cooked side up.

3 Once cooked, remove the pancake from the pan and fry the remaining 2 eggs for 2 minutes until the whites are cooked through but the yolks are still runny.

4 Cut the pancake in half and serve each portion with an egg, lots of sesame seeds, the reserved spring onions and a good glug of hot sauce, if you like.

MANCHEGO + CHORIZO EGG IN A HOLE

Holy moley, Batman. Now that's what I call a breakfast. This is ready in 15 minutes with only a few minutes of prep. Chorizo and Manchego are a Spanish combination well worth getting to know… Delicioso! Feel free to riff on this idea with smoked ham and Gruyère, or salami and Parmesan. All of them are belters.

SERVES 2

2 slices of very thick white bread
10g (¼oz) butter
6 slices of thin chorizo
2 eggs
25g (1oz) Manchego cheese, grated
a pinch of fresh chives, finely chopped
salt and freshly ground black pepper

1 Preheat the oven to 220°C, 200°C fan, gas mark 7.

2 Use the back of a spoon to push down and make an indent in the centre of each piece of bread that's around the same size as a fried egg.

3 Spread the butter over the edges of the bread, then lay 3 chorizo slices per slice of bread along the centre of the indent.

4 Transfer the pieces of bread to a baking tray lined with non-stick baking paper. Crack an egg into the centre of each piece of bread on top of the chorizo, then scatter the Manchego around the edges of each slice – don't be too neat about this; you can deliberately get some on the non-stick baking paper, as this will make a lovely caramelised cheese skirt when it bakes.

5 Stick it in the oven for 10–12 minutes until the egg white is set but the yolk is still runny. It can help to cover the tray with foil for the first 7–8 minutes to kick-start the cooking, depending on your oven, then remove for nice crispy bits.

6 Pull it from the oven, scatter over the chives, season with salt and pepper and enjoy.

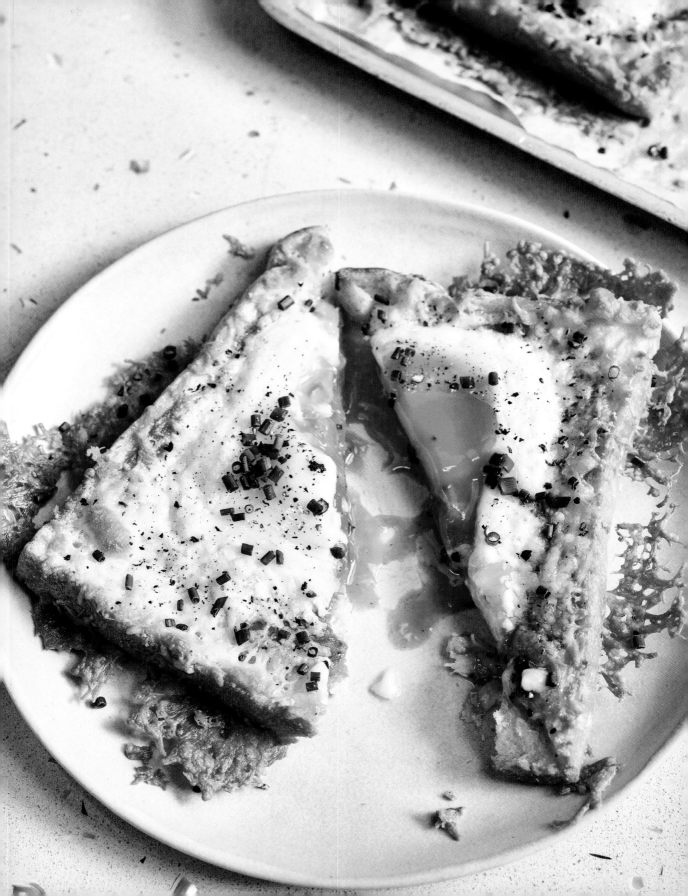

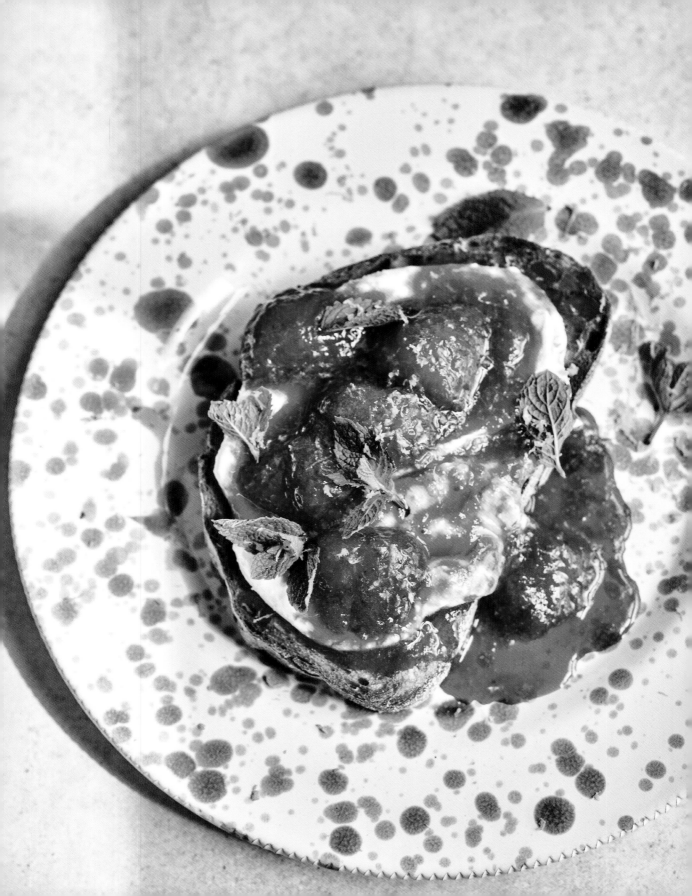

WHIPPED COTTAGE CHEESE + STRAWBERRY COMPOTE TOAST

I know cottage cheese might seem weird – the texture is a bit strange – but blitzing it is a real game-changer. It takes on a new life and tastes really nice and creamy. Cottage cheese is also high in protein and low in fat, and a lovely thing to keep in your fridge. Try putting it on toast with a dollop of pesto and some roasted veggies for a savoury version.

SERVES 2

300g (10oz) strawberries, hulled
2 tbsp caster sugar
zest of 1 lemon, plus 1 tbsp juice
1 tsp vanilla extract
200g (7oz) cottage cheese
2 slices of sourdough
a few sprigs of fresh mint, leaves picked, to serve

1 Add the strawberries to a small saucepan with the sugar, lemon juice and vanilla extract. Cook over a medium heat with the lid on for 5 minutes, then take the lid off and cook for another 6–8 minutes to allow the liquid to evaporate and become syrupy.

2 In the meantime, add the cottage cheese to a blender and blitz until smooth.

3 Toast the sourdough, then top with the whipped cottage cheese. Spoon over some strawberry compote and garnish with the lemon zest and mint leaves.

TIP/SWAP
The compote method here would work with any berry or soft fruit – you can also use frozen fruit.

BLUEBERRY PANCAKES

Blueberry pancakes never get old, and they never go out of fashion. They're a classic at any hotel buffet because everyone loves them. A stack of these always goes down a treat in our house, and adding the sweet, warm blueberry compote seals the deal.

SERVES 4

250g (9oz) blueberries
2 tsp vanilla extract
50ml (2fl oz) water
200g (7oz) natural yoghurt
2 eggs
zest of 1 lemon
2 tbsp vegetable oil
170g (6oz) plain flour
1 tsp baking powder
1 tsp bicarbonate of soda
1 tbsp butter or oil spray
4 tbsp soured cream
maple syrup, to serve
  (optional)

1   Add 150g (5oz) of the blueberries to a small saucepan with 1 teaspoon of the vanilla extract and the water. Bring to a simmer and cook for 5–6 minutes, until the blueberries collapse slightly and the liquid becomes syrupy.

2   In the meantime, add the remaining vanilla to a mixing bowl with the yoghurt, eggs, lemon zest and vegetable oil. Mix well to combine. Add the flour, baking powder and bicarbonate of soda and mix well to combine.

3   Add a little bit of butter to a large frying pan or spray it with oil to lightly coat and heat until the butter is bubbly and the pan is hot. Add 2–3 tablespoons of batter to the pan for each pancake, spaced apart, then dot some blueberries onto the uncooked surface of each. Flip the pancake over after 1–2 minutes when the underside is golden and cooked through, and cook for a further minute on the other side.

4   Serve the pancakes with the blueberry compote and a dollop of soured cream and some maple syrup, if you like.

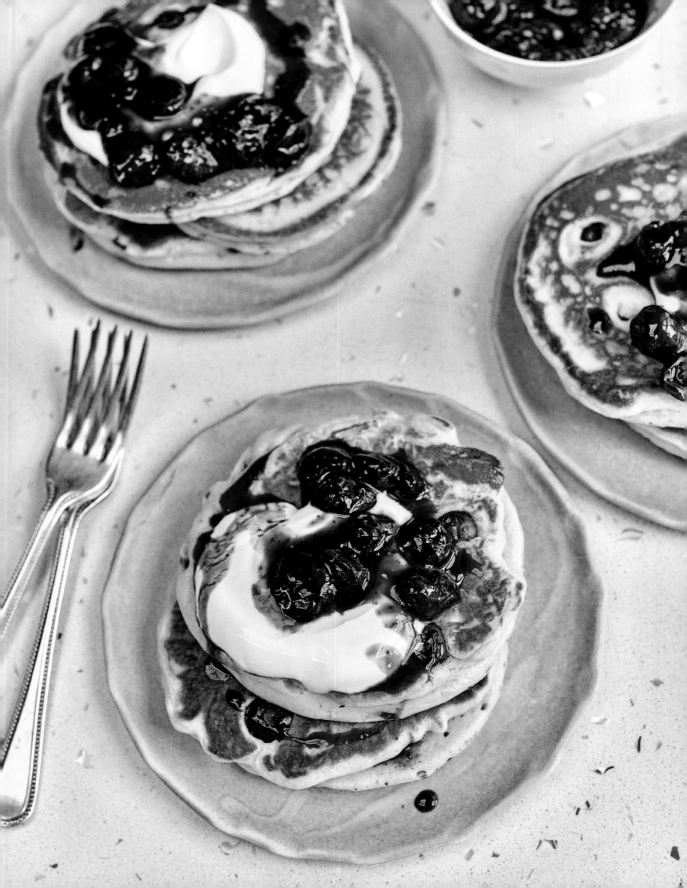

GREEN GODDESS EGGS

I'm obsessed with green goddess salad dressing. If you're not sure what that is or what it tastes like, take my word for it and try this recipe. It tastes so good! I've made this higher in protein by adding some cottage cheese as the base and heaps of herbs and freshness on top. You could definitely do fried or poached eggs with this dish if you wanted. Enjoy!

SERVES 2

2 eggs
1 tbsp olive oil
2 small courgettes, thinly sliced into rounds
handful of spinach or kale leaves (approx. 50g/2oz)
1 avocado, peeled and stone removed
1 garlic clove
2 spring onions, roughly chopped
30g (1oz) mixed fresh soft herbs (I use parsley and coriander)
zest and juice of 1 lemon
100g (3½oz) cottage cheese
2–3 tbsp water
2 flatbreads
50g (2oz) salad, such as watercress or lamb's lettuce
salt and freshly ground black pepper

1 Bring a large pan of water to the boil. Add the eggs and boil for 6½ minutes for jammy eggs. Pour off the boiling water, run under cold water and set aside.

2 Add the olive oil to a large frying pan and fry the courgettes on a medium–high heat until golden, around 3 minutes on each side. Season well with salt and pepper and set aside.

3 Add the spinach or kale, avocado flesh, garlic, spring onions, herbs, lemon zest and juice, cottage cheese and water to a blender. Blitz until smooth and season to taste.

4 Heat the flatbreads directly over the hob using some tongs, or in the toaster.

5 Peel the eggs; it can help to crack the shells on a surface, then peel them under running water – the water gets in between the shell and the egg and loosens everything up.

6 Spoon the green goddess sauce over the flatbreads, and top with the fried courgettes. Slice the eggs in half and place on top. Serve with a handful of salad and enjoy.

TIP/SWAP
Stir a little bit of pesto through the courgettes to take the green flavour to the next level.

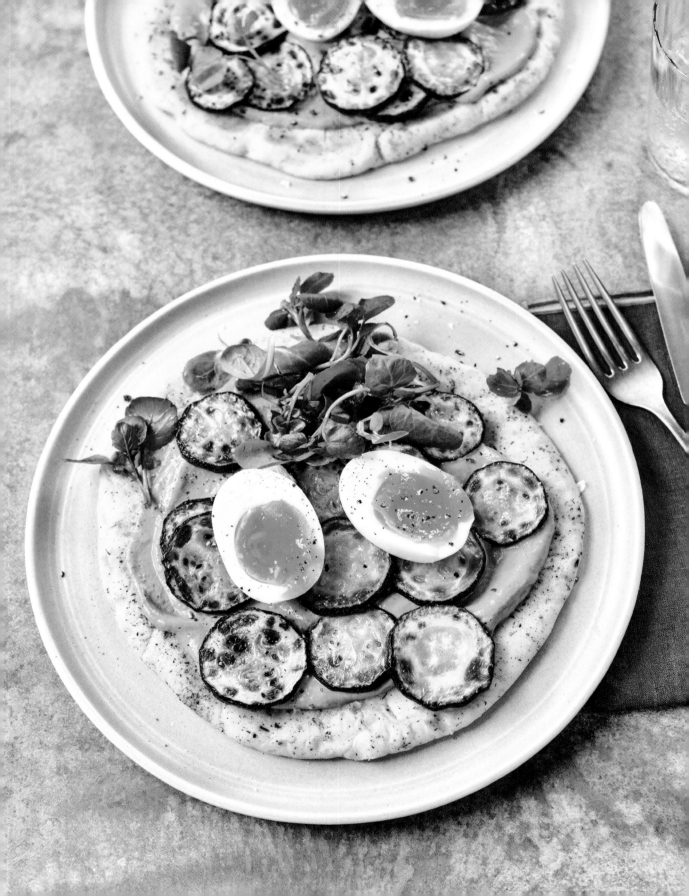

BREAKFAST BRUSCHETTA

What sort of nutter has bruschetta for breakfast? Guilty as charged, Your Honour. Bruschetta is one of the best things on the planet to have, so why don't we have it for brekkie more? This goes down well with a couple of perfectly fried eggs. A winner's breakfast!

SERVES 2

1 ciabatta, cut in half
   horizontally
1 garlic clove, cut in half
2 tbsp extra-virgin olive oil
4 eggs
½ red onion, finely
   chopped
2 tomatoes, chopped
1 avocado, peeled, pitted
   and flesh chopped
a bunch of fresh basil
   leaves, chopped, a few
   small leaves reserved
2 tbsp balsamic vinegar
salt and freshly ground
   black pepper

1 Preheat a non-stick frying pan. Cook the cut side of the ciabatta in the dry pan until it's toasted and golden brown, then rub the cut halves of the garlic clove all over the toasted side of the bread and set aside.

2 Add 1 tablespoon of the oil to the frying pan and crack in the eggs. Fry for 2 minutes until the whites are set and the yolks are still runny.

3 In the meantime, mix the remaining olive oil with the red onion, tomatoes, avocado and basil. Season well.

4 Spoon the bruschetta mixture onto the ciabatta, drizzle with balsamic vinegar and serve with the 2 fried eggs and the reserved basil leaves scattered over.

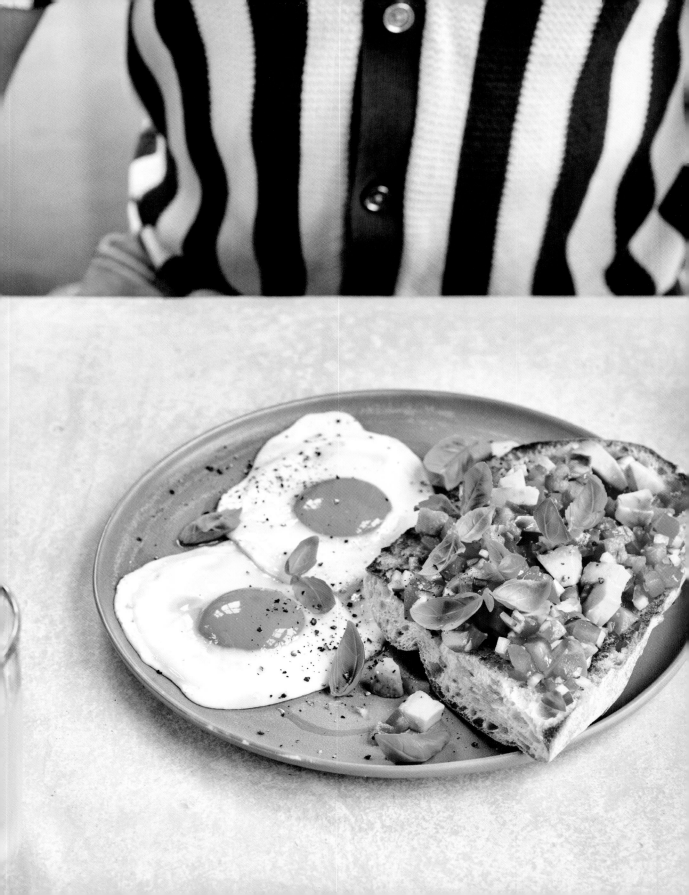

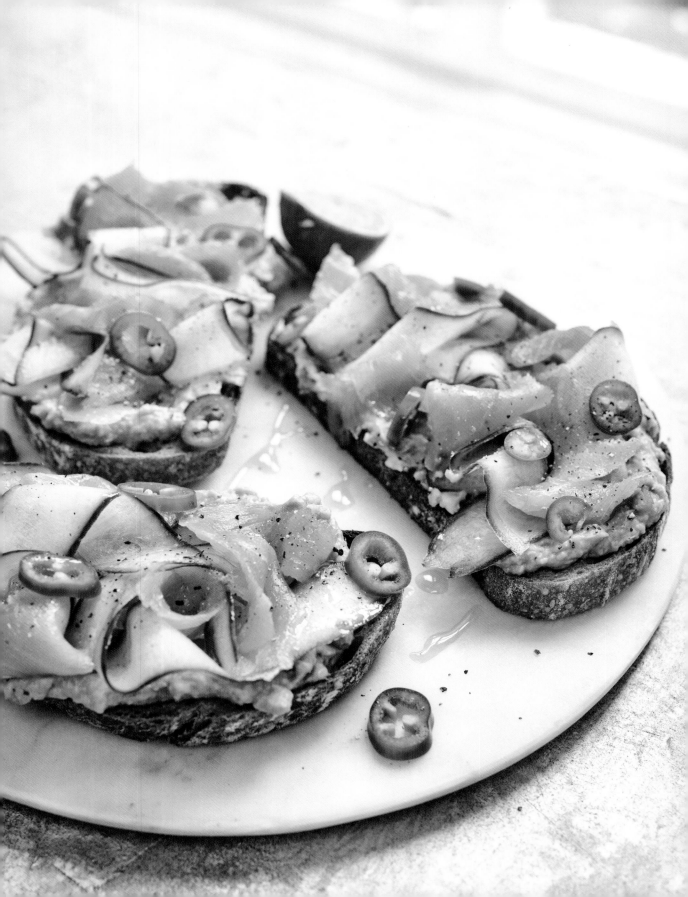

SALMON, AVOCADO + JALAPENO TOAST

Another classic brunch menu option is salmon and avocado on toast. This recipe takes things to the next level with some pickled jalapenos. Blitzing them with avocado makes the most magical avocado crema you will ever taste. Definitely worth a try today.

SERVES 2

2 slices of sourdough
1 avocado
1–2 tbsp pickled jalapenos, to taste
juice of 1 lime
50g (2oz) smoked salmon, sliced into ribbons
¼ cucumber, peeled into ribbons
1 fresh jalapeno or green chilli, thinly sliced (optional)
salt and freshly ground black pepper

1 Pop the sourdough in the toaster and toast for 2 minutes until golden.

2 In the meantime, cut the avocado in half, remove the stone and scoop out the flesh into a blender. Add the pickled jalapenos and lime juice and whizz together in a food processor or blender to a slightly chunky paste. Season well, then spread over the toast.

3 Top with ribbons of smoked salmon and cucumber and extra chilli if using.

HARISSA MUSHROOM, SWEET POTATO + KALE HASH

VG

This is a stonker of a breakfast hash and is ideal for those days you want a healthy veggie option. It's a spicy and amazing savoury option for the morning. The harissa really is the special ingredient in this one, but it could also work well with 2 teaspoons of pesto instead.

SERVES 2

250g (9oz) sweet potato, unpeeled, cut into cubes
2 tbsp extra-virgin olive oil
300g (10oz) baby chestnut mushrooms, halved or quartered
1 red onion, thinly sliced
2 garlic cloves, finely grated or chopped
2 tsp harissa paste
½ bag of kale leaves, shredded
3 roasted red peppers from a jar, sliced into strips
juice of 1 lemon
salt and freshly ground black pepper

1 Pop the sweet potato cubes in a bowl, cover with cling film and microwave for 2–3 minutes until soft.

2 Add the oil to a large frying pan and start to fry the chestnut mushrooms until golden. Chuck in the red onion and fry for 2 minutes until starting to soften.

3 Add the garlic and harissa paste and toss to coat the veg for 2 minutes or until fragrant.

4 Add the softened sweet potato, kale and red peppers and sauté vigorously until the kale has wilted and the sweet potato has gained some colour. Season generously with salt and pepper. Finish things off with a nice squeeze of lemon and enjoy.

TIP/SWAP
If you're not vegan, this would be amazing with a few fried eggs cracked in, shakshuka-style.

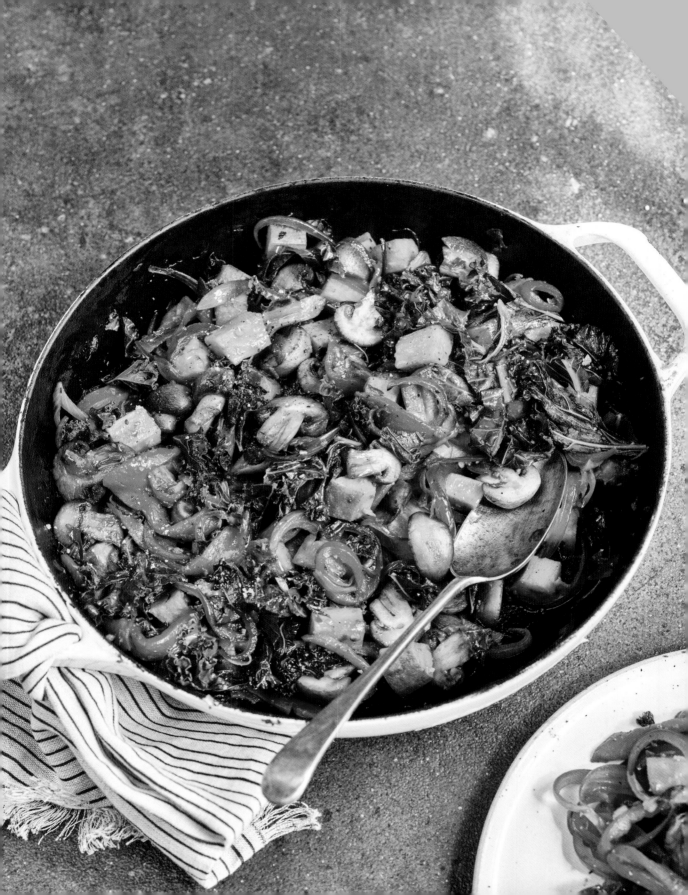

MASALA OMELETTE WITH MANGO CHUTNEY

v

Curry and mango chutney for breakfast? Are you having a laugh? I'll admit it's a bold move, but trust me: it's incredible. You won't want any more boring cheese omelettes after this one. Look at that photo, too. Stunning. This omelette is colourful, full of flavour and perfect for any time of the day.

SERVES 2

½ tsp butter
2 tsp curry paste
1 red onion, finely sliced
100g (3½oz) baby spinach leaves
4 eggs, beaten
30g (1oz) Cheddar cheese, grated
1 tomato, chopped
¼ cucumber, chopped
small handful of fresh coriander, roughly chopped
juice of 1 lime
2 tbsp mango chutney
salt and freshly ground black pepper

1 Add the butter to a medium non-stick frying pan over a medium heat. Once it bubbles, add the curry paste and most of the red onion and cook for 2 minutes until fragrant and starting to soften. Throw in the spinach and allow it to just wilt, then turn the heat right down and pour in the beaten eggs and sprinkle over the Cheddar cheese. Pop a lid on to allow the omelette to cook on top without having to flip it – or you could stick it under the grill for a minute.

2 While the omelette cooks, mix the remaining red onion with the tomato, cucumber, most of the coriander, a big pinch of salt and pepper and the lime juice.

3 Slide the omelette onto a serving platter and top with the salad, mango chutney and the remaining coriander. Slice and enjoy.

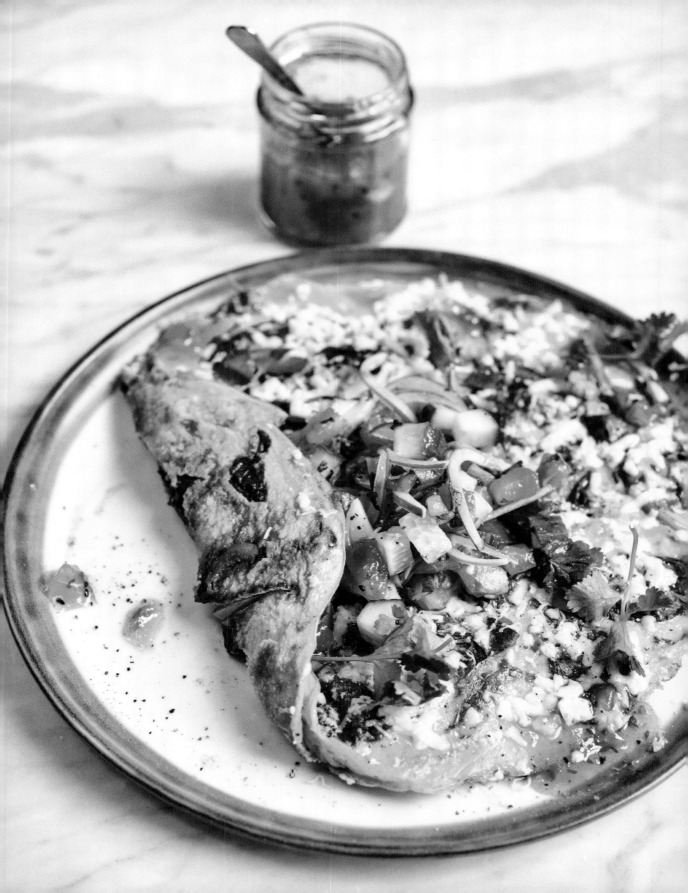

BRULÉE CITRUS BIRCHER

VG

This is one of my go-to breakfasts. It is so simple and easy to make, and adding chopped nuts or seeds gives it a really wonderful crunch. Charring the citrus fruits in a pan gives them a lovely warm and toasty sweetness, but you can also skip this step and enjoy them fresh if you're in a hurry. Just keep half the bircher in the fridge and simply loosen it with a little more milk before you eat it.

SERVES 2

80g (3oz) porridge oats
1 tbsp chia seeds
180ml (6fl oz) soy milk, plus extra to loosen
40g (1½oz) dairy-free yoghurt
1 apple, unpeeled, cored and grated
1 orange, peeled and sliced
½ grapefruit, peeled and sliced

To serve (optional)
handful of chopped nuts, such as almonds, or sunflower or pumpkin seeds
maple syrup

1 Add the oats and chia seeds to a bowl. Mix in the milk, yoghurt and apple. Leave this to sit for 10–12 minutes.

2 Preheat a non-stick frying pan over a high heat. Add the orange and grapefruit slices to the dry pan and char on one side, around 2 minutes. Remove from the pan and set aside.

3 Once the bircher has thickened, you can add a little dash more milk if you like before serving, then top with the charred citrus slices and your favourite nuts or seeds, if using. A small drizzle of maple syrup over it really makes it pop.

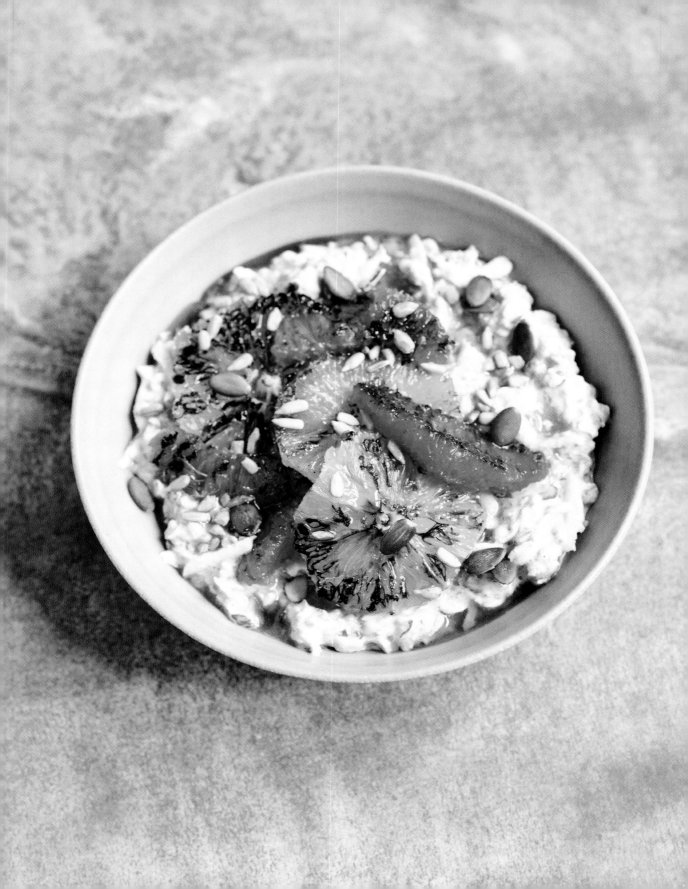

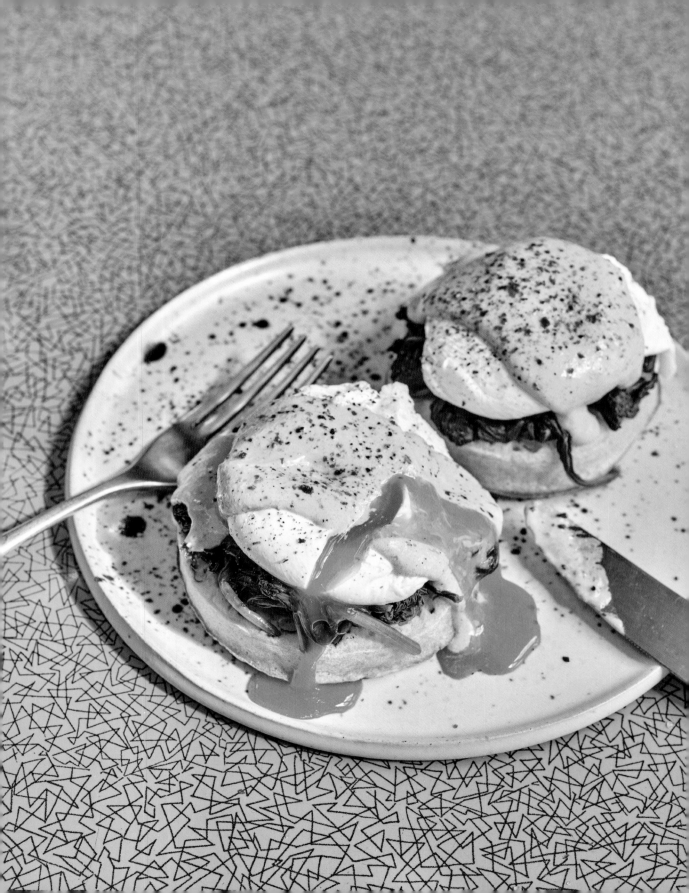

EGGS FLORENTINE

OK, this is not a true hollandaise sauce, complete with half a block of butter – but this yoghurt sauce, flavoured with sun-dried tomatoes and lots of lemon juice, is the perfect alternative and much healthier. We've also swapped English muffins for crumpets to change things up. Hot crumpets are perfect for soaking up all that lovely sauce. Make sure you squeeze as much liquid from your spinach as you can so things don't get soggy. No one likes a soggy bottom!

SERVES 2

150g (5oz) thick Greek yoghurt
50g (2oz) sun-dried tomatoes
juice of 1 lemon
1 tsp hot sauce, plus extra to taste
4 crumpets
1 tbsp white wine vinegar
4 eggs
200g (7oz) baby spinach leaves
½ tsp cayenne or chilli flakes (optional)
salt and freshly ground black pepper

1. Bring a pan of water to the boil. Meanwhile, add the yoghurt, sun-dried tomatoes, lemon juice and hot sauce to a blender with a generous seasoning of salt and pepper. Whizz until smooth and adjust to taste.

2. Get the crumpets in the toaster for 2 minutes. Set aside until you're ready.

3. Add the vinegar to the boiling water and turn the heat right down to a bare simmer. Crack the eggs directly into the water to poach – don't worry about whirlpools or any other faff; they'll still taste great even if they've got wispy bits of whites. For runny yolks you'll only need to cook the eggs for about 2 minutes – use a slotted spoon to get them out and poke the yolk with your finger, and if it feels bouncy and not jelly-ish, they're ready.

4. In a separate dry pan, wilt the spinach – alternatively, you can do this in the microwave if you don't want to get another pan dirty! Once it's wilted, tip it into a sieve and squeeze out any excess moisture. Season well.

5. Serve the spinach on top of the crumpets, topped with a poached egg and a decent spoonful of the yoghurt sauce. Finish with a nice sprinkle of cayenne or chilli flakes, if you like, and tuck in.

CHIPOTLE FRITTATA LOADED BAGELS

WOW! Look at that photo and tell me you don't wanna 'av a bang of that. I mean, come on. It's ridiculous. I could eat both of them right now. If you love a classic egg and bacon sarnie, then this posh version with the spicy frittata, crispy bacon and hot sauce is going to blow you away. Absolutely magnificent beast. Go on, get stuck in!

MAKES 2, WITH LEFTOVER FRITTATA

oil spray
6 eggs
2 tbsp milk
1 tbsp chipotle paste
3 spring onions, finely sliced
½ red pepper, deseeded and finely chopped
½ green pepper, deseeded and finely chopped
large handful of fresh coriander, finely chopped
4 rashers of back bacon
2 bagels, sliced in half horizontally
2 slices of cheese (optional)
8 sun-dried tomatoes
handful of baby spinach leaves
hot sauce, to serve
salt and freshly ground black pepper

1 Preheat the oven to 200°C, 180°C fan, gas mark 6. Grease a small baking dish with oil spray.

2 In a medium bowl, whisk the eggs with the milk, chipotle paste, spring onions, peppers and coriander and season generously. Pour this mixture into the baking dish and transfer to the oven for 8–10 minutes until puffed up and set with no visible runny egg.

3 In the meantime, get your bacon in a frying pan and cook over a medium heat for 3 minutes on each side until nice and golden.

4 Toast the bagels in the toaster, or just toast the cut sides in the bacon pan.

5 Layer up each bagel base with a slice of cheese, if you like, some sun-dried tomatoes, bacon and baby spinach leaves. Slice the frittata into 6 squares and lay one square on top of each of the bagels (saving the rest as leftovers). Load up with hot sauce and enjoy.

TIP/SWAP

If you have an air fryer and your dish fits inside the drawer, you can also whack the frittata in there for 8 minutes at 200°C, 180°C fan, gas mark 6, or until set.

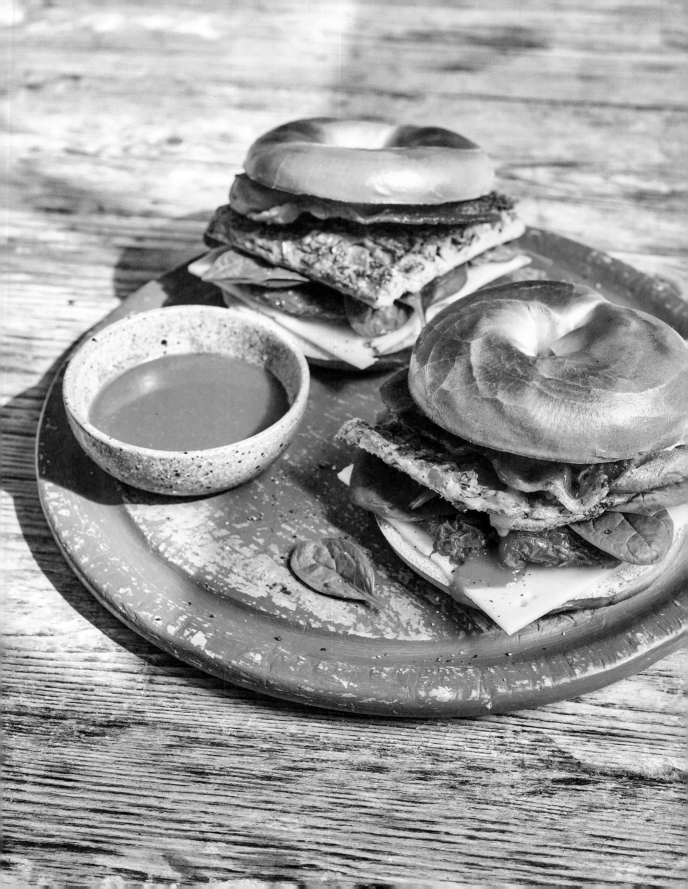

LUNCH

Lunch doesn't have to be the same old boring sandwich meal deal or bland salad eaten in a rush at your desk. You can cook and prepare delicious recipes at home which are varied, full of flavour and properly nutritious to energise yourself and make you feel good during the day. I believe in trying to make things that taste great hot and fresh but also eaten cold on the go too.

There are plenty of great options to choose from here, which you will love to make over and over again. The key thing for sticking to a healthy diet is, I believe, meal prepping and being in control of what you eat. If you leave the house with one of these delicious lunch recipes, you are defending yourself against the world of fast food and ultra-processed convenience foods on the go. This is how you stay on track. This is how you win! Good luck. You can do it!

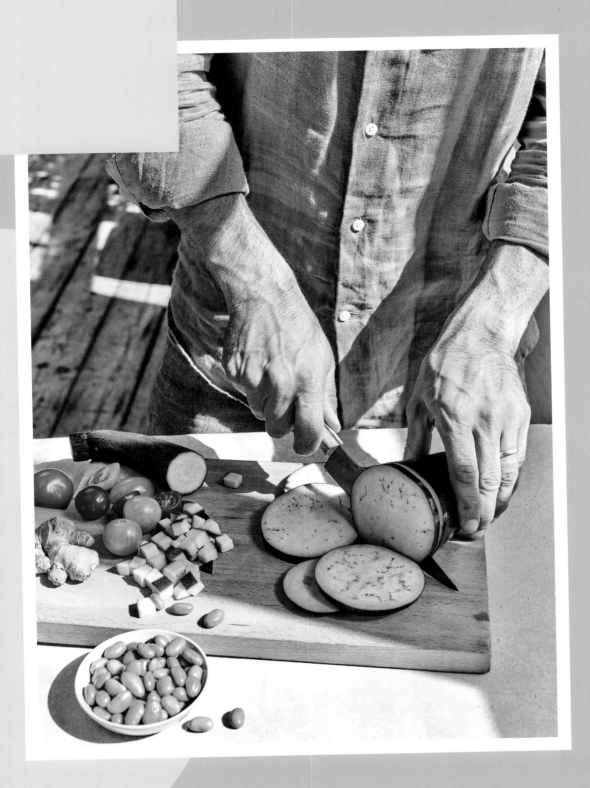

HARISSA PRAWN COUSCOUS BOWL

This is a beautiful Mediterranean take on a poke bowl. Lots of fresh flavours with a hit of spicy harissa paste on the prawns. This is a dream lunch and can be enjoyed hot or cold, so is perfect for when on the go.

SERVES 2

150g (5oz) cherry tomatoes
120g (4½oz) couscous
165g (5½oz) raw king prawns
1 tbsp harissa paste
4 tbsp olive oil
5 sprigs of fresh tarragon, plus extra to garnish
3 sprigs of fresh mint, plus extra to garnish
2 sprigs of fresh oregano, plus extra to garnish
juice of 1 lemon, divided
2 tbsp balsamic vinegar
100g (3½oz) fresh edamame beans
¼ cucumber, sliced
salt and freshly ground black pepper

1 Pop the tomatoes into a dry non-stick frying pan and cook for 10–12 minutes, until charred and bursting.

2 Get the kettle on, then pour the couscous into a bowl and cover with boiling water. Throw a tea towel on top, or use cling film to cover, and set aside for 10 minutes.

3 In the meantime, marinate the prawns with the harissa paste, 1 tablespoon of the oil and a pinch of salt.

4 Finely chop all of the herbs and add half of them to a small bowl with the remaining olive oil, half the lemon juice and the balsamic vinegar.

5 When the couscous is tender, add the remaining chopped herbs and lemon juice and season with salt and pepper.

6 Remove the tomatoes from the pan and fry off the prawns while the pan is nice and hot – they should get a lovely char and turn pink through by cooking for 1 minute on each side.

7 Serve the prawns and tomatoes on a bed of herby couscous with the edamame and cucumber slices. Pour over the dressing, garnish with your herbs and enjoy.

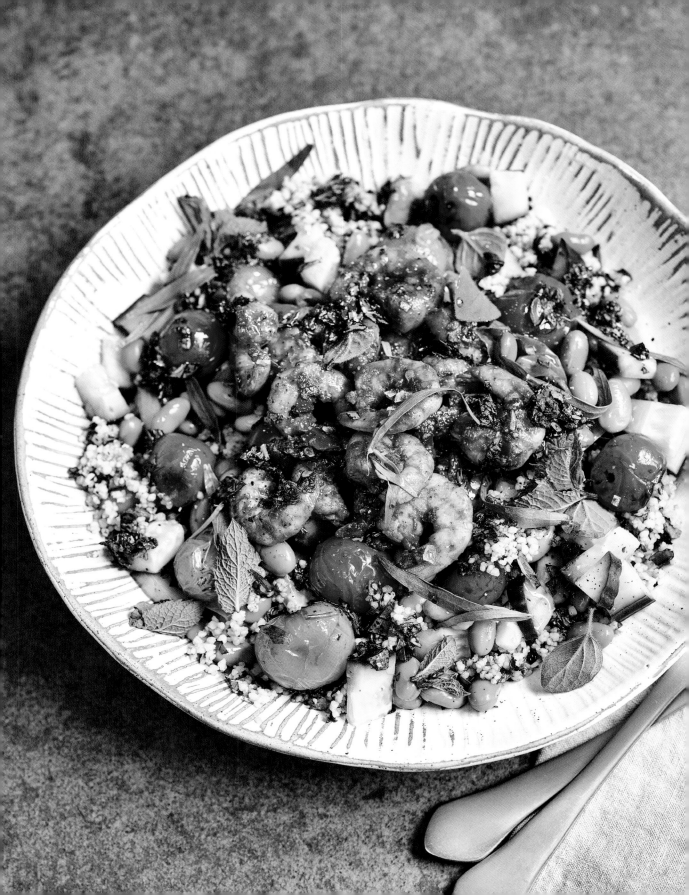

CACIO E PEPE BEANS 'N' GREENS

Oh hello, Captain Farty Pants! Fancy some more beans? This is probably one of the stranger-looking recipes in this book, but don't judge it on its looks alone, because this cheesy dish tastes magnificent and it's another great one for the all-important gut health.

SERVES 2

1 tbsp extra-virgin olive oil
1 shallot, finely chopped
4 garlic cloves, grated or finely chopped
400g (14oz) tin of butter beans
½ tbsp freshly ground black pepper
40g (1½oz) Parmesan, finely grated, plus extra to serve
1 tbsp red wine vinegar
150g tender stem broccoli
100g kale

1 Get the kettle on.

2 Heat the oil into a deep frying pan, then sauté the shallot for 2–3 minutes until softened, stirring regularly. Add the garlic and fry for 1 minute until fragrant, then throw in the tin of butter beans, along with any liquid from the tin. Bring up to a simmer, add the pepper, Parmesan and red wine vinegar. Don't skimp on the pepper here – it's the main flavour, and you want it to be almost spicy.

3 Pour the boiling water into a saucepan and boil the broccoli and kale for 2–3 minutes until tender. Drain, season well and set aside.

4 Serve the beans in two bowls, topped with broccoli and kale with a little bit of extra Parmesan.

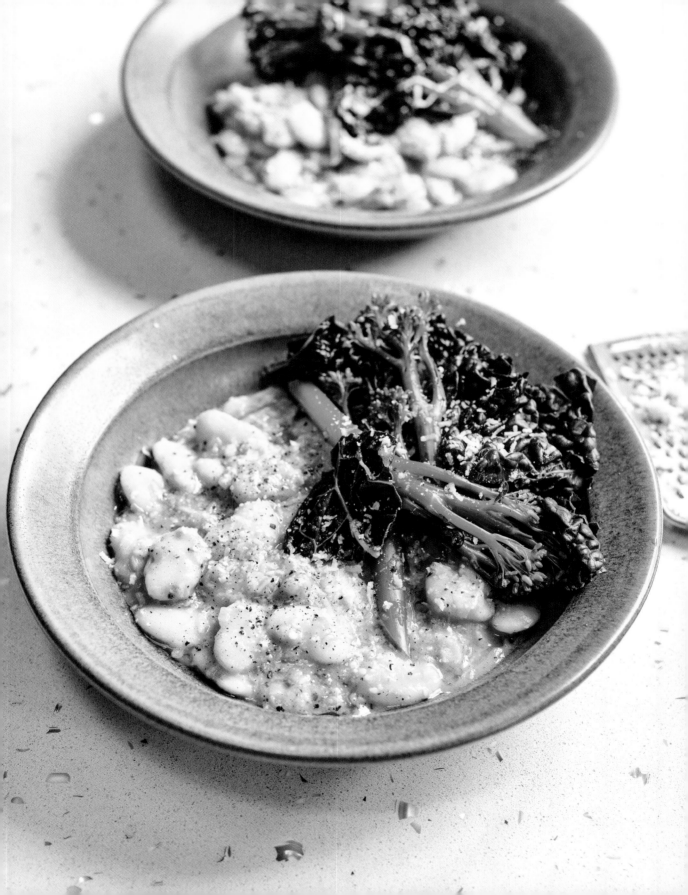

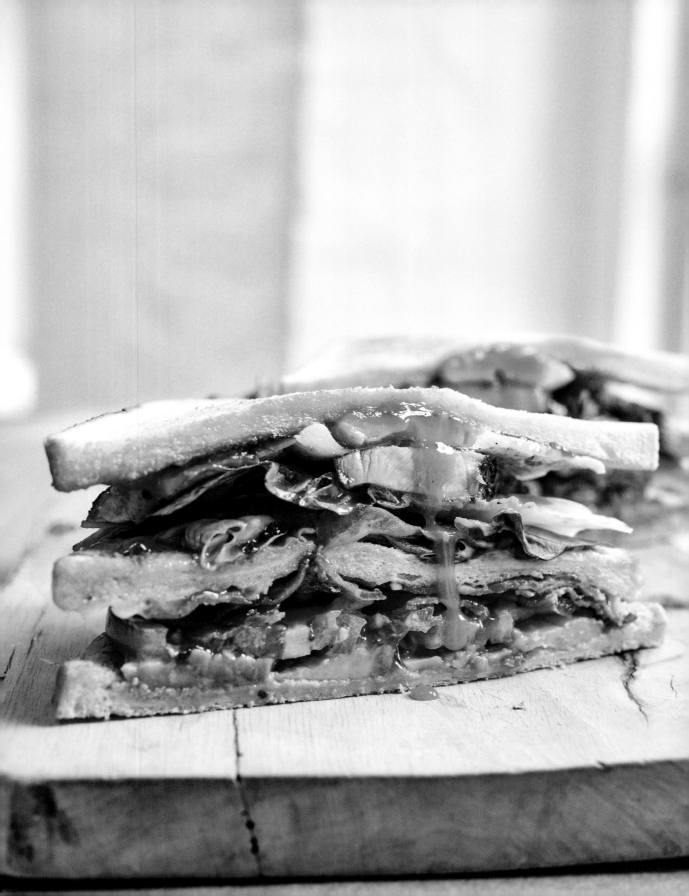

CHILLI CHICKEN CLUB SANDWICH

Corrr, yes please – I'd like to join this club! Three slices of bread in a sandwich is madness, but it's also kind of genius, isn't it? Look at it. Layers for days. You'd need a big old mooey to get this one down you in one bite. It's got a double spice kick from the chipotle paste and chilli jam. My biggest tip is to use a bread knife to slice through it to make sure you keep everything intact.

MAKES 1

½ tsp chipotle paste
1 chicken breast
2 slices of streaky bacon
1 egg
3 slices of bread
1 tbsp mayonnaise
2 tbsp chilli jam
½ avocado, peeled, stone removed and sliced
juice of ½ lime
½ tomato, sliced
4 Little Gem lettuce leaves
salt and freshly ground black pepper

1 Rub the chipotle paste all over the chicken breast and sprinkle it with salt and pepper – if it's a particularly fat one, use a knife to make a slit in the fattest part so you can open it out and it cooks faster. Preheat a frying pan and dry-fry the chicken and bacon in the same pan until the bacon is crisp and the chicken is cooked through – you shouldn't need any oil because the bacon will release its fat.

2 Remove the chicken to a plate to rest, then fry the egg in the chicken and bacon juices until the white is set and the yolk is still runny, about 1½ minutes.

3 Get the bread in the toaster. Once toasted, spread the mayonnaise on one side of the bread. Spread the chilli jam on another slice. Lay the avocado slices on the last piece of toast and mash lightly with a fork, then season with the lime juice, salt and pepper.

4 Starting with the avocado toast, top with the tomatoes and bacon. Lay the mayonnaise slice on top, followed by the chicken, egg and lettuce. Sandwich the layers together with the chilli jam toast. Slice in half and enjoy.

HALLOUMI + FALAFEL BOWLS WITH QUINOA

It doesn't get much fresher than this. This is a bit like a loaded tabbouleh salad – totally customisable and great for a fridge raid. You can just chuck in any salad bits that you like. Easy and delicious!

SERVES 2

3 tbsp tahini
4 tbsp water
1 tsp maple syrup
juice of 1 lemon
250g (9oz) pouch of prepared quinoa
30g (1oz) flat-leaf fresh parsley, finely chopped
15g (½oz) fresh basil, finely chopped
15g (½oz) fresh mint, finely chopped
½ red onion, finely chopped
150g (5oz) cherry tomatoes, chopped
¼ cucumber, chopped
400g (14oz) tin of chickpeas, drained and rinsed
1 red pepper, deseeded and chopped
1 tbsp olive oil
1 packet of halloumi, cut into 8 slices
4 falafels (approx. 100g)
80g (3oz) pomegranate seeds
30g (1oz) pistachios, chopped
salt and freshly ground black pepper

1 In a small bowl, whisk the tahini, water, maple syrup and half the lemon juice. Season to taste and set aside.

2 Empty out the quinoa into a large mixing bowl and pour in the remaining lemon juice. Mix with the parsley, basil, mint, red onion, cherry tomatoes, cucumber, chickpeas and red pepper. Season to taste.

3 Add the oil to a large non-stick frying pan and fry the halloumi until golden, around 1 minute on each side.

4 Divide the quinoa salad between two bowls and top each with 4 slices of halloumi, 2 falafels and a sprinkle of pomegranate seeds and pistachios. Drizzle with the tahini dressing and enjoy.

TIP/SWAP
You can do this with just falafels to make this a vegan dish.

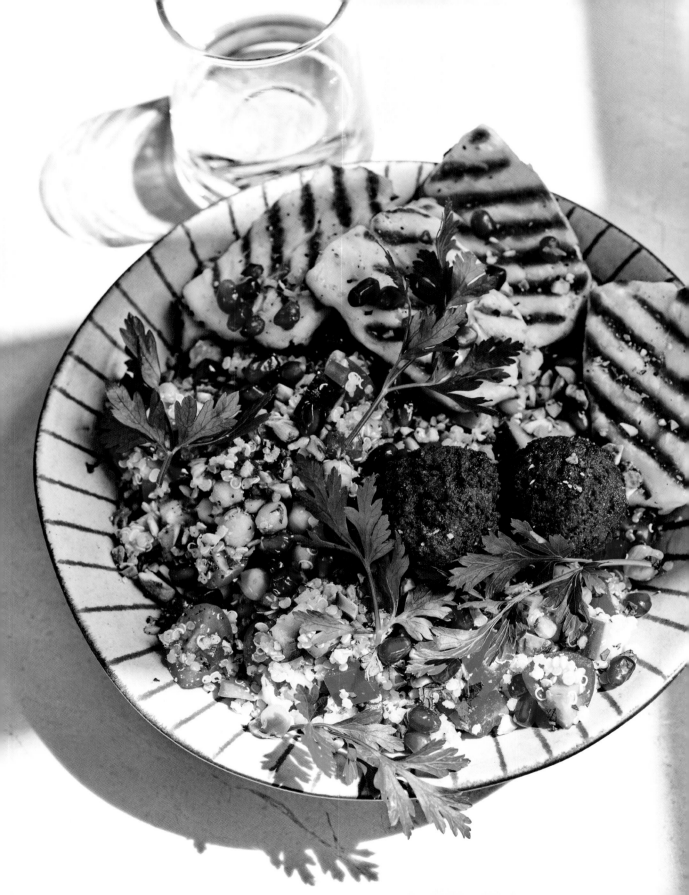

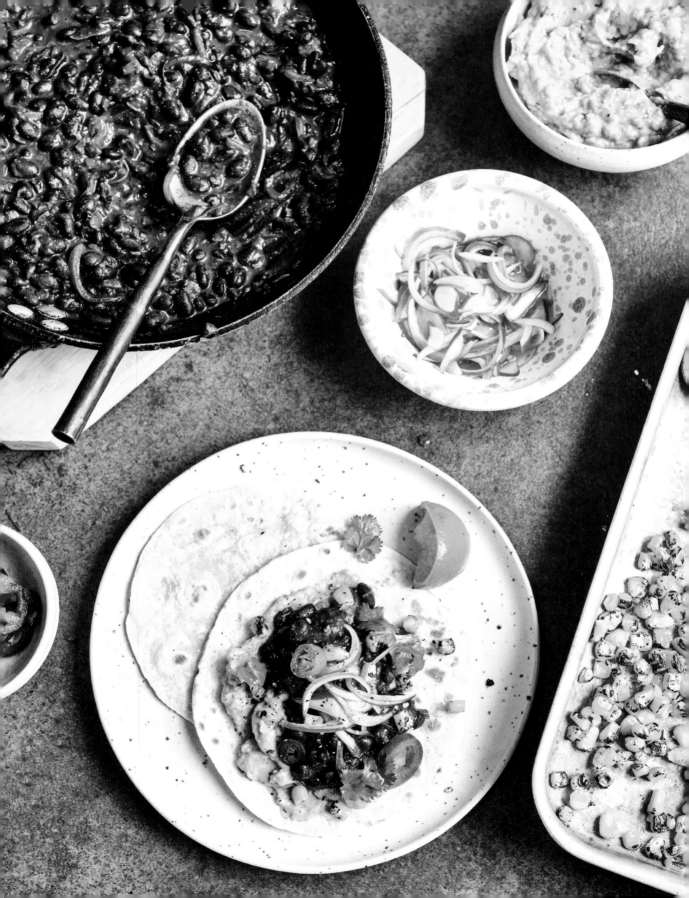

BLACK BEAN TACOS

Full of protein, full of flavour, full of beans! This quick avocado crema is so easy – just blitzing together avocado with lime juice and coriander makes an amazing condiment to have on hand. Store it in the fridge covered with cling film (make sure the cling film is directly touching the surface of the cream to stop it from going brown).

SERVES 2

1 red onion, thinly sliced
2 limes
1 tbsp extra-virgin olive oil
4 garlic cloves, grated or finely chopped
1 tbsp chipotle paste
1 tbsp ground cumin
400g (14oz) tin of black beans
6 small corn tacos
2 avocados, peeled and stone removed
small handful of fresh coriander
200g (7oz) tin of sweetcorn, drained
2 tbsp pickled jalapenos (optional)
salt and freshly ground black pepper

1 Put half of the onion into a bowl with the juice of half of one of the limes and a big pinch of salt. Scrunch the slices to coat them in the juice and set aside to lightly pickle.

2 Put the remaining onion into a frying pan with the olive oil and fry for 2 minutes until softened. Add the garlic, chipotle paste and cumin and cook for 1 minute until fragrant.

3 Add the black beans along with the liquid from the tin – this will help the sauce to thicken up fast, but if you don't like the idea of the bean liquid, just add a big splash of water instead.

4 While the beans are bubbling away, warm the corn tacos in the microwave or over the gas flame directly using tongs to get a bit charred.

5 Scoop the avocado flesh into a blender with most of the coriander, the juice of one lime and a pinch of salt. Blitz until smooth.

6 To serve, add a heaped tablespoon of black beans to the taco, and top with corn, the pickled onions, avocado crema and some pickled jalapenos, if you like things spicy. Slice up the remaining lime half and serve the wedges alongside for an extra tangy hit.

→ TIP/SWAP

You can dry-fry the corn in a pan to char it for an extra flavour dimension if you like – or just eat it as is.

HARVEST GRAIN BOWL

Eating your 5-a-day has never been easier. Heaped with vegetables and smothered in a herby soured cream ranch dressing, this is the perfect all-year-round salad. It makes great use of those bags of pre-chopped squash or sweet potato you find in the supermarket – of course you can chop your own but buying them ready-prepped is a real time saver on busy days.

SERVES 2

½ red onion, thinly sliced
juice of 2 lemons
100g (3½oz) kale, finely
   shredded
100g (3½oz) Brussels
   sprouts, finely shredded
1 tbsp extra-virgin olive oil
½ a 400g (14oz) packet of
   pre-cut butternut squash
300g (10oz) soured cream
½ bunch of fresh chives
½ bunch of fresh parsley
½ bunch of fresh dill
1 garlic clove
250g (9oz) grain pouch of
   your choice
1 apple, cored and diced
30g (1oz) pecans, roughly
   chopped
30g (1oz) dried cranberries
salt and freshly ground
   black pepper

1 Add the onion to a small bowl with the juice of half a lemon and a big pinch of salt. Scrunch the slices in your hands to coat them in the juice, then set aside to lightly pickle.

2 Toss the shredded kale and Brussels sprouts with the juice of 1 lemon, the oil and plenty of salt and pepper. Massage with your hands for 1 minute to tenderise the leaves, then set aside.

3 Put the butternut squash into a microwave-safe bowl, cover with cling film and microwave on high for 5 minutes or until tender.

4 In the meantime, add the remaining lemon juice to a blender with the soured cream, chives, parsley, dill and garlic. Blitz until smooth and season to taste.

5 To assemble the salad, divide the grain pouch among two bowls and top with the steamed butternut squash, a large handful of the shredded greens, the apple chunks, chopped pecans and dried cranberries. Drizzle with the dressing and enjoy.

TIP/SWAP
A little bit of crumbled blue cheese or goat's cheese over the top here would go so well.

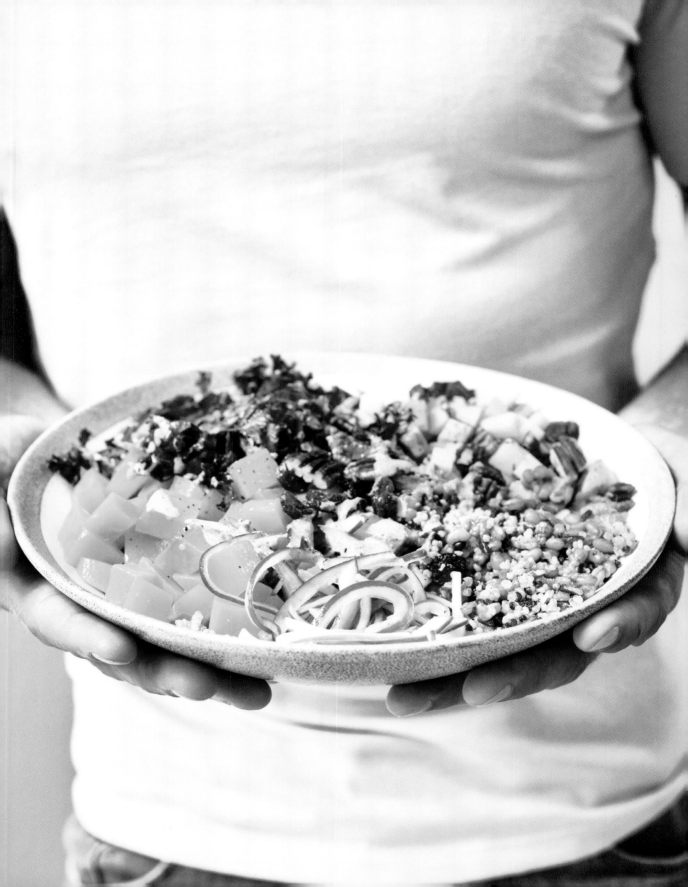

NACHO BEEF BURRITOS

These burritos ditch the rice to load up on fresh salad and crunchy tortilla crisps, so this ends up tasting like a gorgeous plateful of nachos, all wrapped up conveniently in a burrito sleeping bag. This makes too much beef mince for two burritos, but it's great to keep prepped in the fridge for another meal. It will keep in the fridge for up to 3 days, or alternatively you can freeze it – just make sure to defrost it beforehand and to use it within 3 months.

SERVES 2

1 tbsp olive oil
500g (1lb 2oz) beef mince
2 tbsp fajita seasoning
1 red pepper, deseeded
  and thinly sliced
½ red onion, finely chopped
1 tomato, finely chopped
1 avocado, peeled, stone
  removed and finely
  chopped
small handful of fresh
  coriander, finely chopped
½ Little Gem lettuce,
  shredded
juice of 1–2 limes
2 tbsp soured cream
2 extra-large tortilla wraps
35g (1½oz) Cheddar
  cheese, grated
2 handfuls of tortilla chips
salt and freshly ground black
  pepper
hot sauce, to serve

1 Add the oil to a large frying pan and tip in the mince. Fry for 3–4 minutes until golden, breaking it up well with the back of a wooden spoon, then add the fajita or taco seasoning, red peppers and 2 tablespoons of water. Fry until the peppers have softened slightly, then turn off the heat.

2 Mix together the onion, tomato, avocado, coriander and Little Gem lettuce. Season with lime juice and salt, set aside.

3 Spread 1 tablespoon of soured cream on each tortilla wrap, sprinkle over the Cheddar cheese and a few spoonfuls of the salad mixture, then top with some beef and red onions. Crumble a handful of tortilla chips on top, then fold in the corners and tightly roll up into a burrito, taking care to keep everything tucked in.

4 Heat a dry frying pan and toast the burrito on all sides until crisp and golden and enjoy with lots of hot sauce.

TIP/SWAP
It helps to microwave the tortilla wraps for 30 seconds before rolling to make the wrap more malleable.

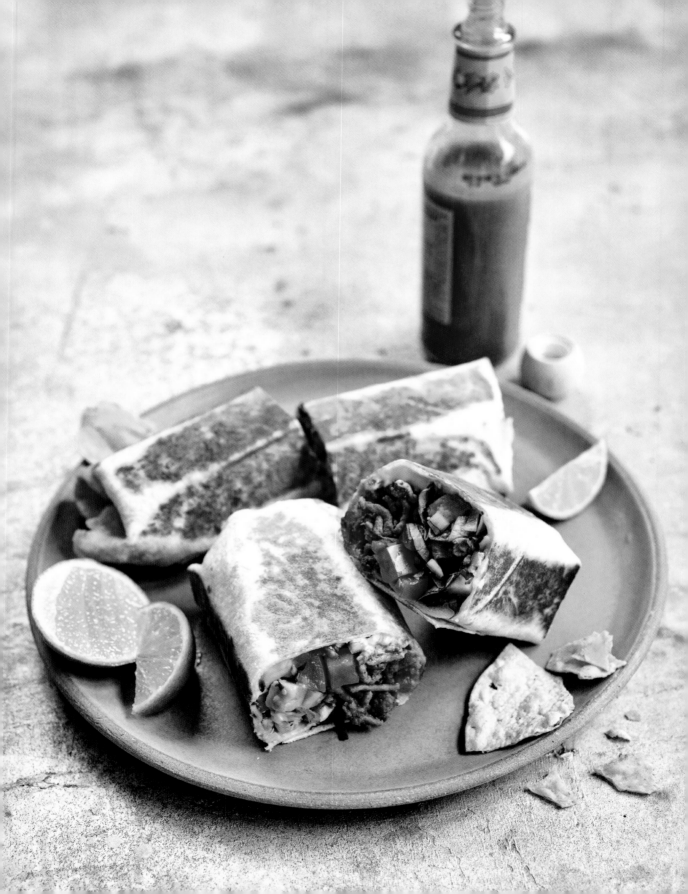

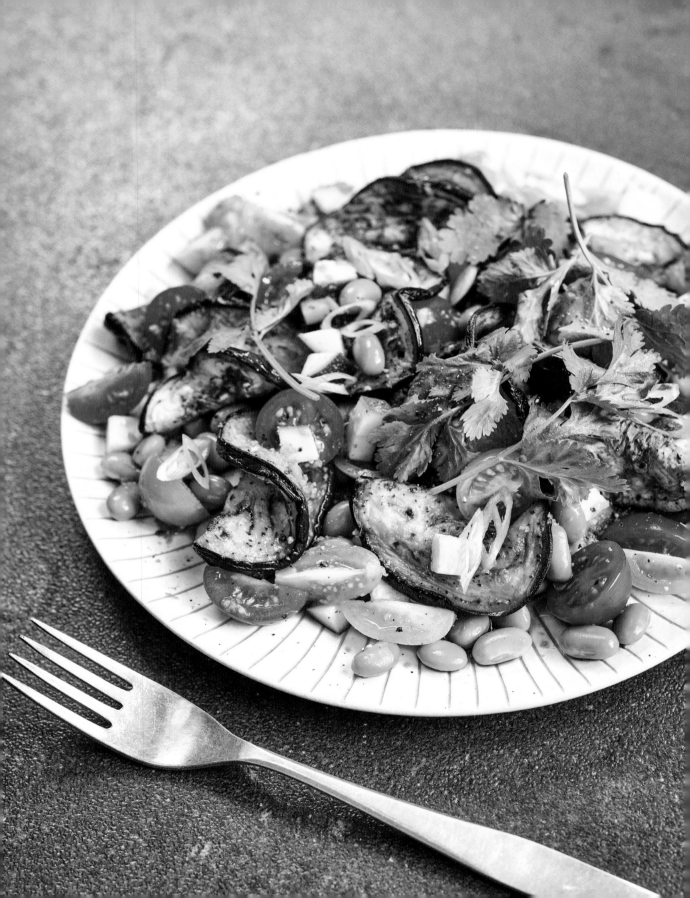

SOY AUBERGINE + COURGETTE SALAD

VG

This salad is summer in a bowl – you've never had anything like it. Plus, if you've never tried raw courgette, you're in for a treat – it's crisp and so nice to eat, with a lovely soy flavour. You can also swap the edamame for broad beans when they're in season. This is great for lunch on the go.

SERVES 2

2 tbsp olive oil
1 aubergine, sliced into 1cm (½in) rounds
1 courgette, finely diced into 5mm (¼in) cubes
175g fresh edamame beans
300g (10oz) ripe tomatoes, halved, sliced or cut into chunks depending on size
2 spring onions, thinly sliced
3 tbsp soy sauce
2 tbsp rice vinegar
thumb-sized piece of fresh ginger, peeled and grated
fresh coriander leaves, to garnish

1 Heat a large frying pan, then add in 1 tablespoon of the olive oil. Arrange the aubergine slices in a single layer and fry until soft and deeply golden, around 3 minutes on each side. You may need to do this in batches; if so, use the extra tablespoon of olive oil depending on the size of your pan and aubergines.

2 In the meantime, toss together the courgette, edamame beans, tomatoes, spring onions, soy sauce, rice vinegar and ginger. Set aside to marinate.

3 When the aubergine is cooked, quickly toss through the salad and serve with coriander leaves to garnish.

PISTACHIO PESTO GNOCCHI SALAD

Pesto is one of my store-cupboard staples, but sometimes it needs a little boost. Adding extra basil, spinach and pistachios to shop-bought pesto takes it to another level. This is delicious served straight away or it works perfectly boxed up for a picnic. Cooking the green beans and the gnocchi in the same pan saves time and washing up.

SERVES 2

150g (5oz) green beans, trimmed
2 tbsp pesto
40g (1½oz) pistachios, roughly chopped
20g (¾oz) fresh basil leaves, plus extra to garnish
50g (2oz) spinach leaves
zest and juice of 1 lemon
2 tbsp olive oil
250g (9oz) packet of gnocchi
200g (7oz) cherry tomatoes, cut in half
100g (3½oz) rocket
225g (8oz) mozzarella pearls (125g/4½oz drained weight)
salt and freshly ground black pepper

1 Get a large pan of water on to boil. Season the water well with water, then throw in the green beans. Set a timer for 5 minutes.

2 In the meantime, add the pesto, most of the pistachios, basil, spinach, lemon zest and juice along with 1 tablespoon of the olive oil to a blender and blitz until smooth. Season to taste and set aside.

3 After 5 minutes, add the gnocchi to the pan of boiling water and beans – wait until they rise to the surface, around 2 minutes, then drain the beans and gnocchi together.

4 Toss the gnocchi and green beans with the pesto and arrange on a platter with the cherry tomatoes, rocket and mozzarella and scatter with the remaining pistachios and the extra basil leaves. Drizzle with the rest of the olive oil and enjoy.

TIP/SWAP

Some sun-dried tomatoes in this would be fabulous if you have them knocking around. Also feel free to swap the gnocchi for any pasta, or even butter beans for a lower-carb version.

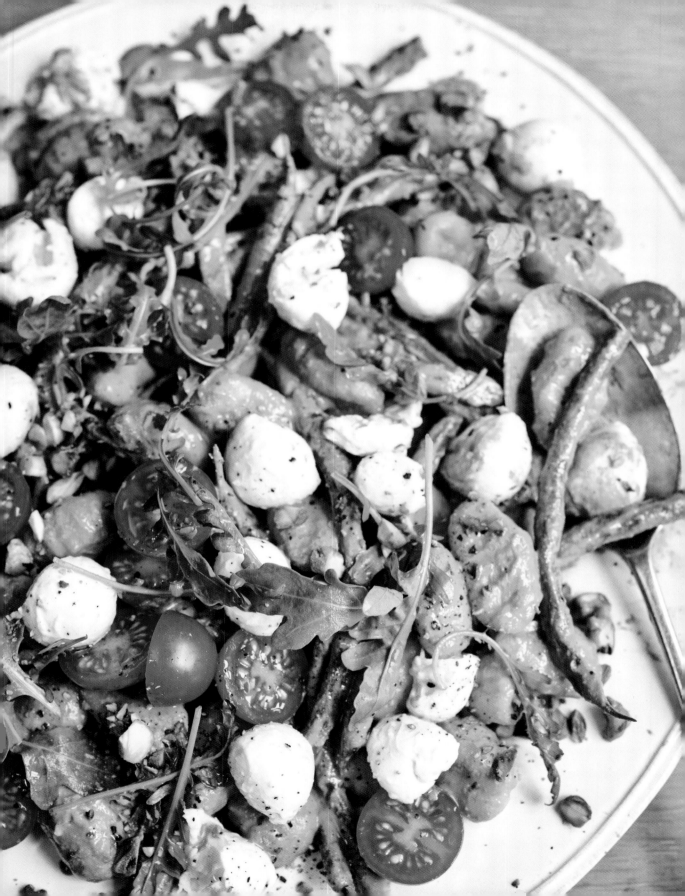

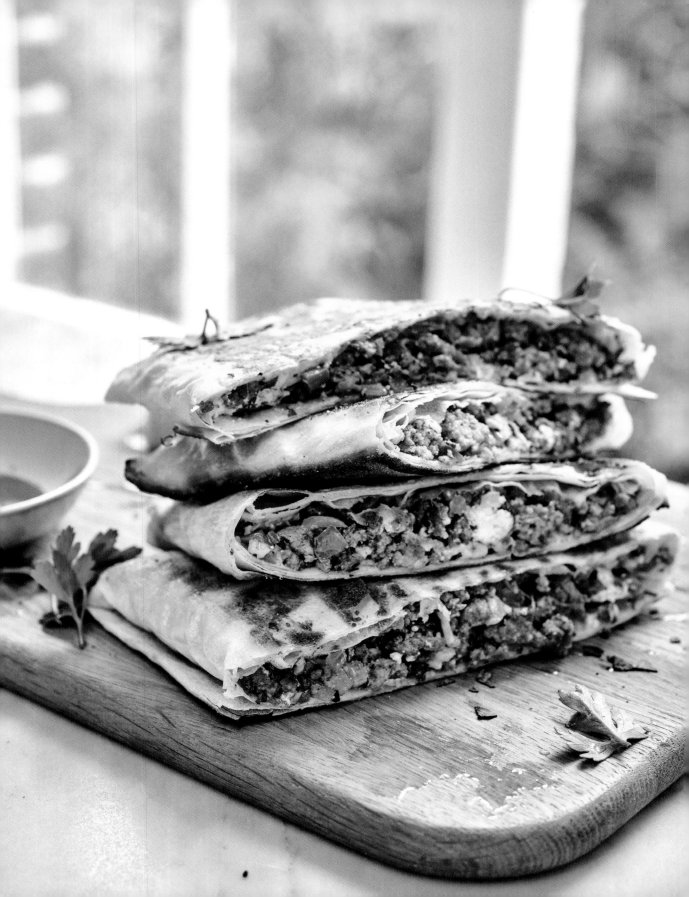

BEEF + FETA FILO PIES

These little pan-fried filo parcels are so much fun to whip up. Inspired by Turkish gözleme, they're great for meal prep, too, as they can easily be reheated in the oven or air fryer. Note that in fifteen minutes you're most likely to get only two pies fried off and ready to eat, but the leftover filling can be stored for another time – otherwise get two pans on the go to have all of them ready together!

MAKES 4

1 tbsp olive oil
500g (1lb 2oz) beef mince
1 onion, finely chopped
1 green pepper, deseeded and finely chopped
2 tbsp ras el hanout
100g (3½oz) feta cheese, crumbled
100g (3½oz) mozzarella cheese, grated
large handful of fresh flat-leaf parsley, finely chopped (30g bunch)
juice of 1 lemon, plus wedges to serve
8 sheets of filo pastry
1 egg, beaten
oil spray
salt and freshly ground black pepper
hot sauce or chilli jam, to serve

1 Heat the olive oil in a large frying pan, then add the beef mince and cook for 2 minutes until browned – pour away any water that collects, then add the onion and green pepper and fry over a high heat for another 2–3 minutes.

2 Add the ras el hanout, fry for 1 minute, then remove from the heat. Season generously with salt and pepper and add the crumbled and grated cheese, along with most the parsley, reserving some for garnish. Squeeze over half the lemon juice.

3 Lay out 2 sheets of filo pastry on top of each other, covering the remaining filo sheets with a damp tea towel to stop them drying out before you need them. Place a small rectangle of filling in the centre, leaving a large border around the edge. Fold the four corners of the first piece of filo over the filling so all the filling is hidden. Flip the parcel over onto the other sheet of filo, then fold over the four corners of that piece of filo – this should ensure no rips or tears of filling will seep through. Brush the side that is visible on top with the beaten egg.

4 Heat another frying pan with a few squirts of oil spray, then fry the filo parcel egg-wash side down. While it is frying on the first side, brush the remaining side with the egg.

5 Make the other parcels while the filo is frying – it should take 1–2 minutes on each side to become crisp. Keep the first batch warm while you cook the last two pies.

6 Enjoy with lots of hot sauce or chilli jam, the remaining parsley scattered over and a squeeze more lemon juice.

SALMON MANGO POKE BOWL

A poke bowl makes lunch feel almost effortless – you do all your chopping in advance, then mix and match with your favourite toppings throughout the week. All of the ingredients included here are optional, so feel free to customise – the dressing goes well with any kind of poke bowl. You're going to want to look out for sushi-grade salmon here, but all fishmongers should have it.

SERVES 2

250g (9oz) sachet of sticky rice
2 tbsp rice vinegar
3 tbsp soy sauce
1 tbsp sesame oil
juice of ½ lime
1 garlic clove, grated
thumb-sized piece of fresh ginger, grated
1 chilli, finely chopped (optional)
120g (4½oz) sushi-grade salmon, cut into cubes
½ mango, peeled, stone removed and chopped into cubes
large handful of fresh edamame beans
¼ cucumber, sliced
⅛ red cabbage, shredded
½ carrot, grated
2 radishes, thinly sliced

1 Microwave the rice pouch, then tip into a bowl and stir through the rice vinegar. Set aside to cool.

2 In a small bowl, mix together the soy, sesame oil, lime juice, garlic, ginger and chilli. Set aside.

3 Divide the rice between two small bowls, then top with the salmon, mango, edamame beans, cucumber slices, shredded cabbage, grated carrot and radishes.

TIP/SWAP

If you're not close to a fishmonger or don't like the idea of eating raw fish, you can cube the fish and fry it in 1 tablespoon of olive oil until it turns opaque and golden, then continue with the recipe as normal.

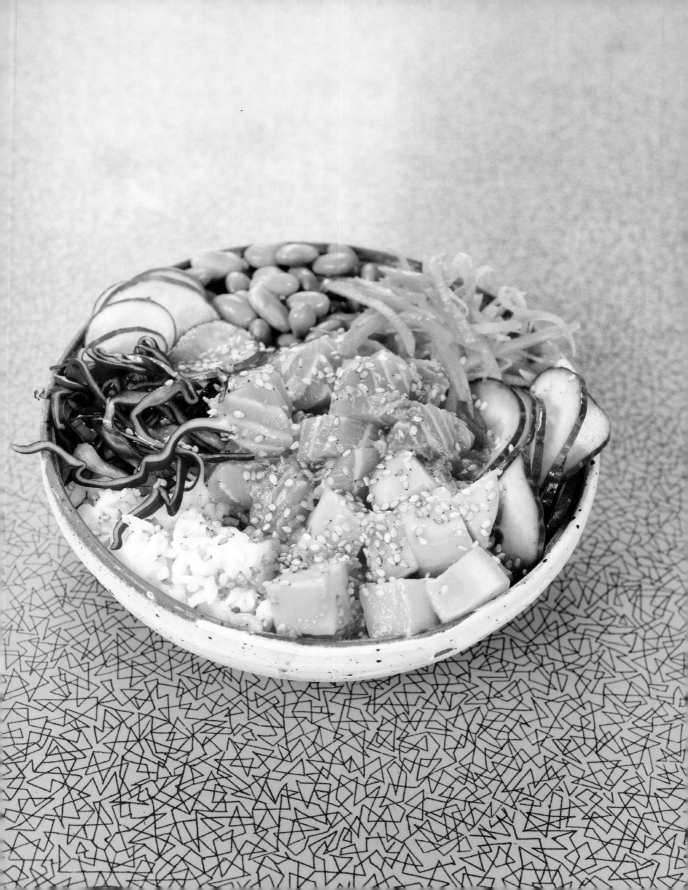

CHICKPEA + TOMATO STEW

This Mediterranean-style stew is so comforting and insanely quick to rustle up. Grating halloumi is a game-changer – it's sharp and tangy and melts beautifully on top of the stew. You are going to enjoy!

SERVES 2

2 tbsp extra-virgin olive oil
1 leek, finely sliced
2 courgettes, cut into 2cm (¾in) dice
1 large baking potato, cut into 1cm (½in) dice
3 garlic cloves, finely grated
2 tsp dried oregano
400g (14oz) tin of chickpeas, drained and rinsed
400g (14oz) tin of chopped tomatoes
500ml (18fl oz) vegetable stock
zest and juice of 1 lemon
100g (3½oz) halloumi, grated
salt and freshly ground black pepper

1 Heat a large saucepan or casserole dish over a medium heat. Add the oil, leek, courgettes and potato and fry for 2–3 minutes until the leek starts to soften.

2 Add the garlic and the oregano and fry for 1 minute or until fragrant.

3 Pour in the chickpeas, chopped tomatoes and vegetable stock and season well. Bring up to the boil, then reduce to a medium simmer for 12 minutes or until the potatoes and courgettes are tender. Season with lemon zest and juice.

4 Spoon into bowls and top with the grated halloumi.

TIP/SWAP
Without the halloumi, this is a fantastic vegan dish.

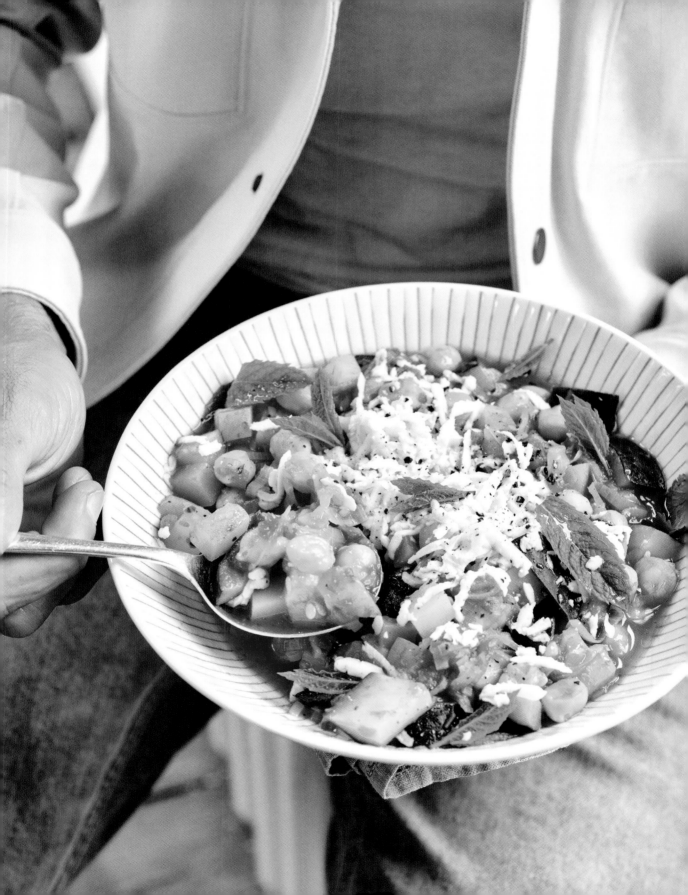

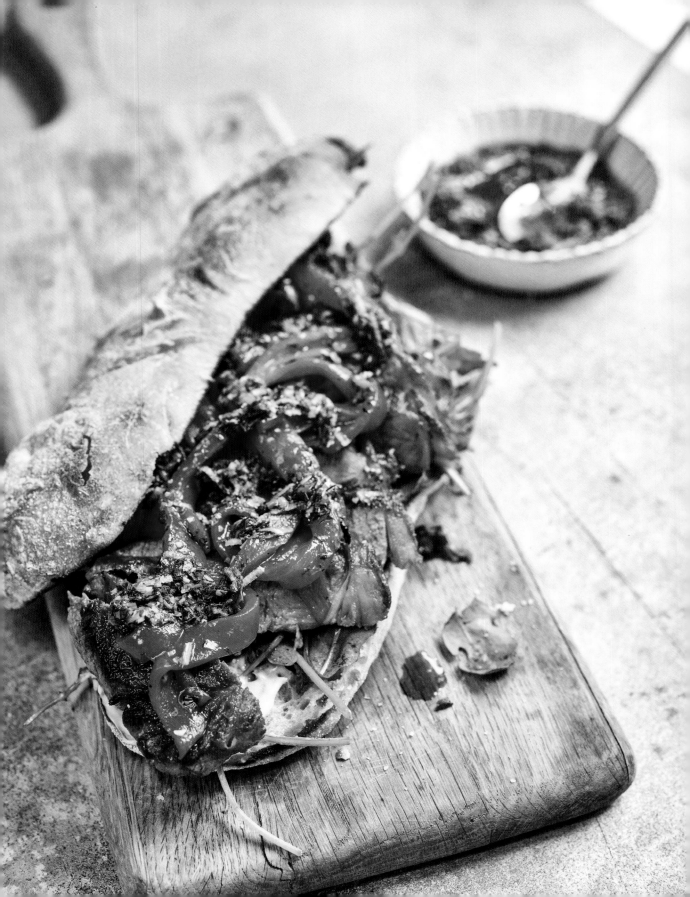

CHIMICHURRI STEAK SANDWICH

Chimi who? Chimichurri. I can't get enough of the stuff. And look at that photo. Is that not the best-looking steak sarnie you've ever seen? Go on, you know you wanna get your laughing gear round that.

SERVES 2

2 steaks of your choice
  (sirloin or rump work well)
5 tbsp olive oil, plus 1 tsp
3 tbsp red wine vinegar
bunch of fresh parsley, finely
  chopped
4 garlic cloves, finely
  chopped
2 tsp chilli paste or 1 chilli,
  finely chopped, with or
  without seeds
1 tsp dried oregano
1 ciabatta
2 tbsp mayonnaise
3 roasted red peppers from
  a jar, sliced into strips
2 large handfuls of rocket
salt and freshly ground black
  pepper

1 Pat down the steaks with kitchen paper, then salt them and rub all over with 1 teaspoon of olive oil. Preheat a frying pan over a high heat.

2 For the chimichurri, mix together the remaining olive oil, red wine vinegar, parsley, garlic, chilli paste and oregano. Season to taste – it should be sharp, fragrant and spicy.

3 Add the steak to the frying pan and cook undisturbed for 2–3 minutes on the first side until you get a good char, then flip and cook for a further minute for a medium–rare steak. Set aside on a chopping board to rest.

4 Slice the ciabatta horizontally and toast each piece cut side down in the hot pan until crisp.

5 Spread the mayonnaise on the bottom of the ciabatta and top with the roasted red peppers and sprinkle with the rocket. Slice up the steaks and lay on top, then slather with the chimichurri. Put the top of the ciabatta on, then split the ciabatta in two to serve.

LAARB SALAD

This salad is quick, easy and bursting with flavour. Absolutely anyone you make this for is going to love it. My kids really enjoy it, too. The dressing is so yummy and will work with chicken, turkey, pork or beef – any kind of mince is delicious.

SERVES 4

1 tbsp vegetable oil
500g (1lb 2oz) chicken mince
4 tbsp lime juice
3 tbsp soy sauce
4 garlic cloves, finely chopped
2 lemongrass sticks, finely sliced
2 shallots, thinly sliced
4 lime leaves, thinly shredded
2 heads of Little Gem lettuce, leaves separated
1 carrot, julienned (or very thinly sliced into batons)
1 cucumber, julienned (or very thinly sliced into batons)
5 radishes, thinly sliced
15g (½oz) fresh mint leaves
15g (½oz) fresh coriander leaves

For the tamarind dressing
3 tbsp tamarind sauce
3 tbsp lime juice
1 shallot, finely chopped
1 chilli, finely chopped
salt and freshly ground black pepper

1 Start by gathering your ingredients and doing your chopping so everything is ready to toss in.

2 Heat the vegetable oil in a large frying pan, add the chicken mince and break it apart well with a wooden spoon so it is in very small, crumb-like pieces. Once the chicken has turned white and begun to gain a little bit of golden colour, splash in the lime juice and soy sauce with the garlic. Fry for 1 minute until little liquid remains in the pan.

3 Turn off the heat and stir through the lemongrass, sliced shallots and lime leaves.

4 Mix together the ingredients for the dressing in a small bowl – season to taste.

5 Shred or rip the lettuce leaves into the bottom of a serving bowl, top with the julienned carrot and cucumber. Spoon over the chicken mixture and top with the radish slices and lots of herbs, then drizzle over the dressing.

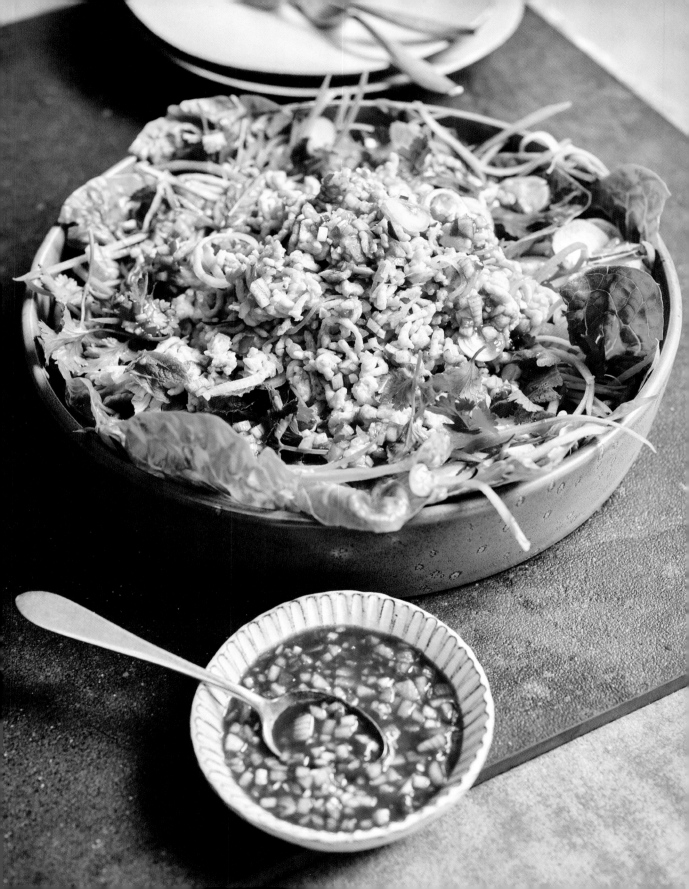

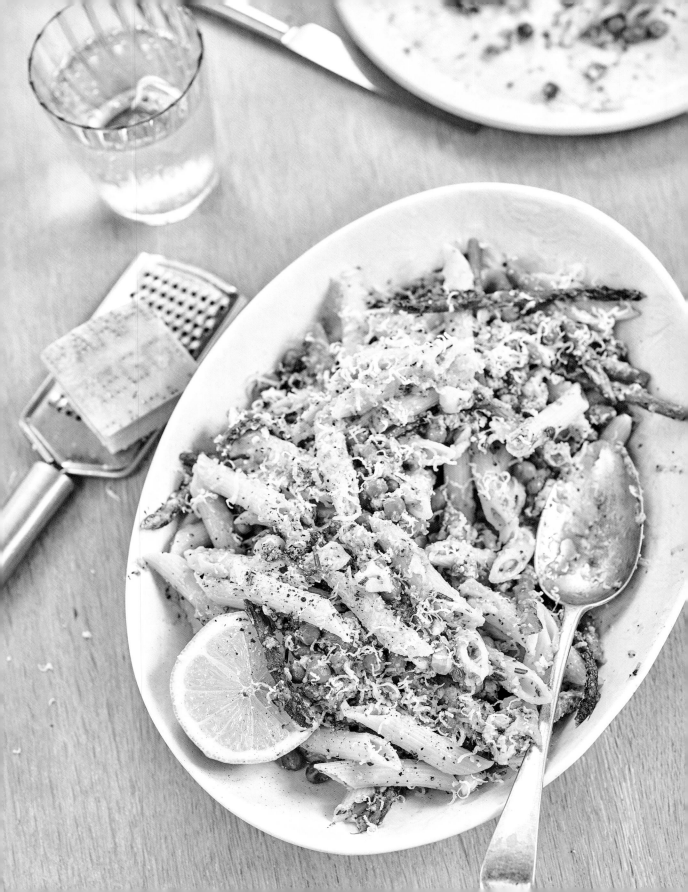

SPRING VEGETABLE PASTA

If health is wealth, then get this recipe off the shelf, you elf. The crisp asparagus, the sweet burst of peas, the super-soft broccoli that coats the pasta almost like a pesto – this dish is absolutely banging. The trick is to cut the broccoli quite small, as you're going to intentionally overcook it – you will love it when it all mixes in with the pasta.

SERVES 4

1 head of broccoli, finely
   chopped, stalk discarded
300g (10oz) penne pasta
2 tbsp extra-virgin olive oil
200g (7oz) asparagus, cut
   into 2–3cm (¾–1¼in)
   chunks
4 garlic cloves, finely
   chopped
4–5 sprigs of fresh rosemary,
   finely chopped
150g (5oz) frozen peas
zest and juice of 1–2 lemons
50g (2oz) Parmesan, finely
   grated, plus extra to serve
salt and freshly ground black
   pepper

1 Stick the kettle on, then pour the boiling water into a large pot. Add the chopped broccoli and penne and boil until the pasta is al dente and the broccoli is very soft, around 9 minutes.

2 In the meantime, in a large frying pan, heat the oil and fry the asparagus until deeply golden and slightly crisp. Throw in the garlic and rosemary and fry for 1 minute until fragrant.

3 Once the pasta and broccoli are cooked, use a slotted spoon to transfer the pasta and broccoli straight into the asparagus pan and toss vigorously with a bit of the pasta water to combine. Add the frozen peas, zest and juice from 1 lemon and the Parmesan and continue to toss vigorously until a glossy sauce clings to the pasta.

4 Plate up with plenty of extra Parmesan for sprinkling.

DINNER

I love food and the way it can bring us all together for a moment. For me dinner time is my favourite meal of the day because it's the time we can all sit together as a family to catch up and laugh about things without being in such a rush. I've created and shared in this chapter what I believe are my best dinner recipes yet. I can always tell how good a recipe is by how many likes, comments and shares it gets on Instagram. All of these were absolute barn burners and went down a storm, so I'm confident you'll enjoy them too.

Again I've tried to include some that are easy to prep with minimum time and also some which can be doubled up and batch cooked for an easier tomorrow with less hassle. There are also a few hacks and tricks to really ensure the recipes will be on your table within 15 minutes. Happy cooking – I hope you enjoy learning new things and building your confidence in the kitchen.

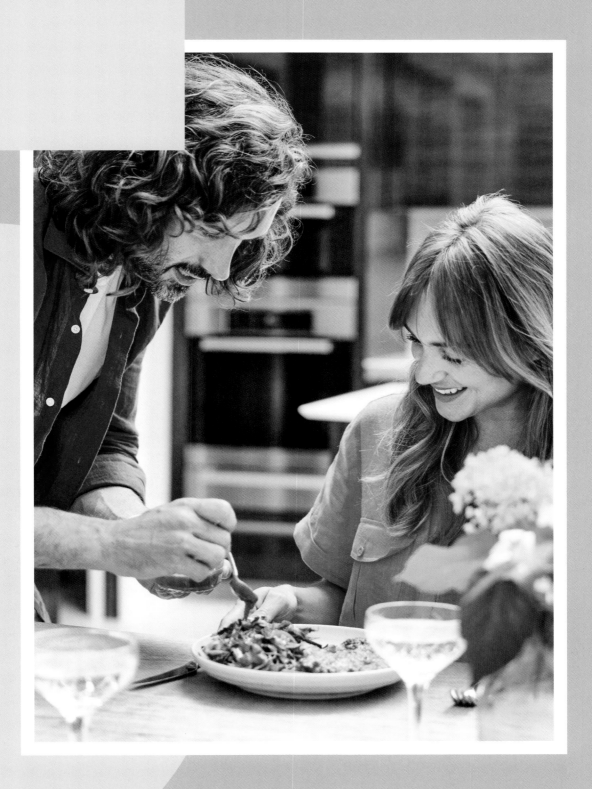

PESTO ORZOTTO WITH AUBERGINES

(VG)

What a beautiful-looking dish this is. If you fancy having a vegan meal tonight, this is perfect. An orzotto is basically a low-maintenance version of a risotto: it has the same gorgeous creamy texture, but it cooks in a fraction of the time. A risotto can sometimes be hard to get right but you can't go wrong with an orzotto.

SERVES 2

vegetable stock cube (to make 750ml–1 litre/ 25–35fl oz stock)
2 tbsp olive oil
2 garlic cloves, sliced or grated
125g (4½oz) orzo
1 aubergine, cut into cubes
150g (5oz) cherry tomatoes
2 tbsp vegan pesto
zest and juice of 1 lemon
salt and freshly ground black pepper
a few sprigs of fresh basil leaves, to garnish
handful of nuts (such as hazelnuts, pine nuts, pistachios), finely chopped, to garnish

1 Stick the kettle on, as you'll need hot vegetable stock soon.

2 Add 1 tablespoon of the oil and the garlic to a frying pan and cook over a medium heat until the garlic wiggles and is fragrant. Throw in the orzo and mix well to coat in the garlic oil, then add 400ml (14fl oz) of the hot vegetable stock and bring to the boil. Stir regularly and keep adding more stock every time the orzo has absorbed the previous batch until the orzo is creamy and cooked through.

3 In the meantime, in another pan, heat the remaining olive oil and fry the aubergine until golden. Add the tomatoes after around 8 minutes of cooking to warm through.

4 Back to the orzotto. Stir through half of the pesto with the lemon zest and juice. Season well to taste.

5 To serve, top with the aubergine and tomato mixture, a little dollop of the remaining pesto, the basil sprigs and chopped nuts.

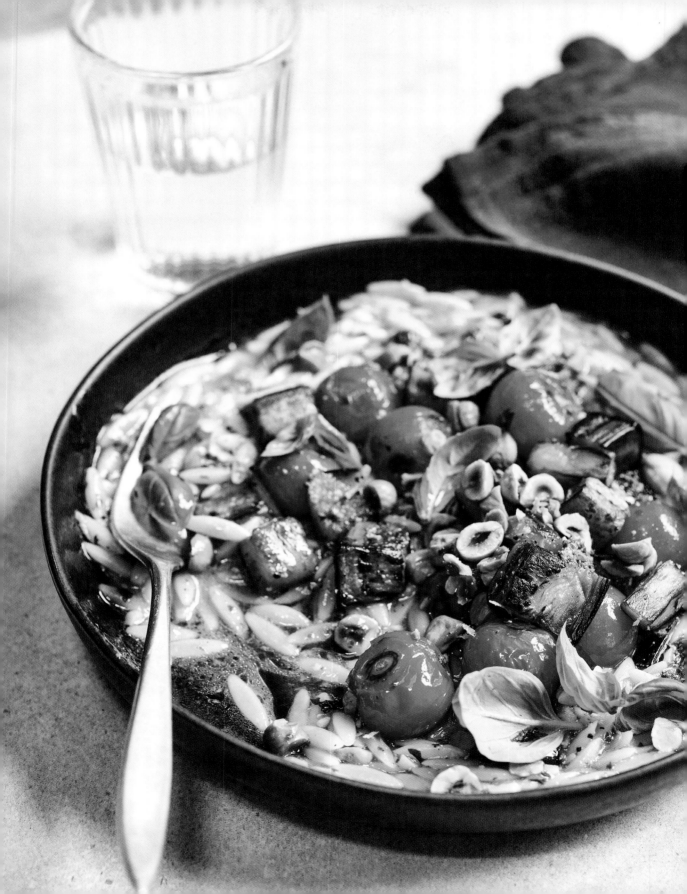

ONION + CABBAGE BHAJI BURGER

VG

Vegan burgers can be dull sometimes, can't they, like eating cardboard. Dry patties? Nah, not for me. But this is without a doubt the tastiest and juiciest vegan burger I've ever got my chops around. I cannot get enough of tamarind sauce – it has an amazing sweet and tangy taste that goes so well with the caramelised onions. Get stuck in. You'll love it, I promise. Cut your onions and cabbage as thin as you can to help it cook through in the short amount of time.

SERVES 2

100g (3½oz) gram flour
1 tbsp garam masala
80ml (3fl oz) water
juice of 1 lime
1 tbsp nigella seeds
1 onion, thinly sliced
¼ Savoy cabbage, thinly
  shredded
2 tbsp vegetable oil
2 vegan burger buns
2 tbsp mango chutney
¼ romaine lettuce,
  shredded
1 tomato, thinly sliced
¼ cucumber, peeled into
  ribbons
handful of fresh mint leaves
3 tbsp tamarind sauce

1   In a medium bowl, whisk together the gram flour, garam masala, water and lime juice until you have a batter-like consistency. Add the nigella seeds, sliced onion and cabbage and toss to coat evenly.

2   Heat the oil in a large frying pan, and once shimmering, divide the batter in two and spoon into the oil in two round patty shapes, pushing down if you need to create a burger-like shape.

3   Fry for around 3 minutes on each side until golden and crisp.

4   Split your buns and spoon mango chutney on the bottom half, then top with lettuce, then a burger, followed by the tomato slices, cucumber ribbons, mint leaves and tamarind sauce. Tuck in.

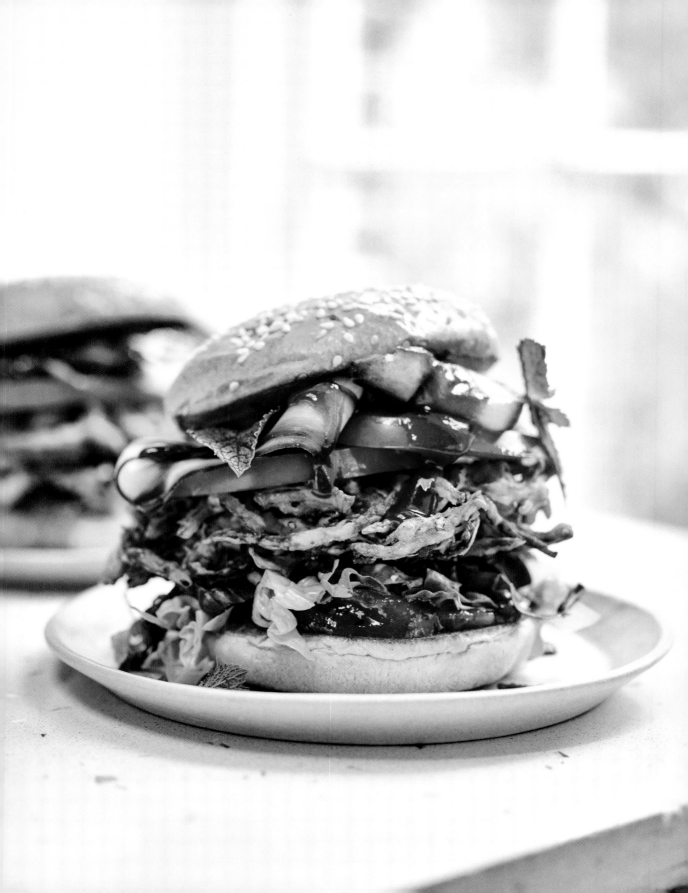

BRISK BANGERS + MASH

Making use of two great hacks here to get dinner on the table in 15 minutes: the microwave and gravy granules, two absolute staples in a British household. Pimping the gravy with a bit of rosemary, balsamic and HP Sauce takes it to the next level. This recipe has a few different things going on at once, so read through it thoroughly before you start to ensure you can get it done in time.

SERVES 4

8 sausages
1 large red onion, thinly sliced
1 tbsp olive oil
500ml (18fl oz) water
400g (14oz) baby potatoes
1 tbsp balsamic vinegar
2 tbsp gravy granules
1 sprig of fresh rosemary, finely chopped
1 tbsp HP Sauce
250g (9oz) Savoy cabbage, finely shredded
1 tbsp salted butter
salt and freshly ground black pepper
½ bunch of fresh chives, finely chopped, to garnish

1 Preheat the grill on its highest setting. Line up the sausages on a tray lined with tin foil and cook, turning them regularly, for 14 minutes until golden and cooked through. Alternatively, air-fry for 12 minutes, turning a couple of times.

2 Next, you'll need to start on the onion gravy. Add the onions to a large frying pan with the olive oil. Cook over a medium heat, stirring regularly and adding a splash of the water every time the pan looks dry or the onions seem to be catching too much colour. This will help them to soften and caramelise faster.

3 In the meantime, pierce the baby potatoes and microwave for 7–8 minutes in a large microwave-safe bowl or until just tender.

4 Once the onions have reduced in volume and cooked down significantly, add the balsamic vinegar and cook for 1 minute until caramelised. Add the gravy granules, the remaining water, rosemary and HP Sauce and allow to bubble up and thicken. Turn off the heat and set aside.

5 Once the potatoes are cooked, crush lightly with the back of a fork, then add the cabbage to the same bowl and microwave again for a further 4 minutes. Stir through the butter and season generously with salt and pepper.

6 Serve the sausages on the cabbage mash with onion gravy and chives sprinkled over.

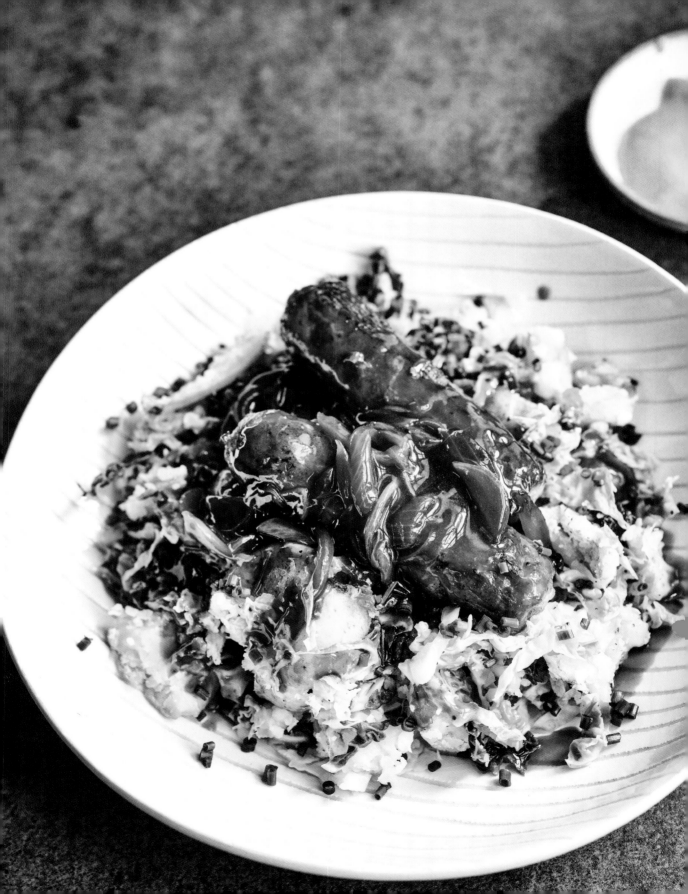

LAMB MEATBALLS, BEETROOT + WHIPPED FETA

Another family favourite in our house. It is just packed with so much flavour! You're going to want to eat the whipped feta with everything, so this deliberately makes a bit too much – keep it in the fridge and thank me later. The yoghurt in these meatballs works to tenderise the lamb really quickly.

SERVES 4

Meatballs
500g (1lb 2oz) lamb mince
50g (2oz) Greek yoghurt
30g (1oz) dried
  breadcrumbs
large handful of fresh
  coriander, finely chopped
2 tbsp harissa paste
1 tbsp olive oil
salt and freshly ground
  black pepper

Whipped feta
200g (7oz) feta
1 garlic clove
100g (3½oz) Greek
  yoghurt

Lentil salad
½ cucumber, cut into cubes
300g (10oz) beetroot in
  vinegar, drained and cut
  into cubes
250g (9oz) pouch of puy
  lentils
100g (3½oz) rocket
squeeze of lemon juice
drizzle of olive oil

1 Preheat the oven to 200°C, 180°C fan, gas mark 6.

2 In a bowl, mix together the lamb mince, yoghurt, breadcrumbs, most of the coriander and the harissa paste. Season generously. Use your hands to mix it all well, then shape into 16 meatballs.

3 Add the oil to a large ovenproof frying pan and fry the lamb meatballs over a high heat for 2 minutes until golden all over, then transfer the frying pan to the oven to allow them to cook through.

4 In the meantime, blitz the feta, garlic and Greek yoghurt in a blender until you have a smooth whipped consistency. Add some cold water, tablespoon by tablespoon, to make it more of a drizzly dressing.

5 For the salad, toss together the cucumber, beetroot, lentils and rocket and give it a big squeeze of lemon juice and a drizzle of olive oil.

6 Serve the meatballs on top of the lentil salad with lots of whipped feta dressing and the reserved coriander.

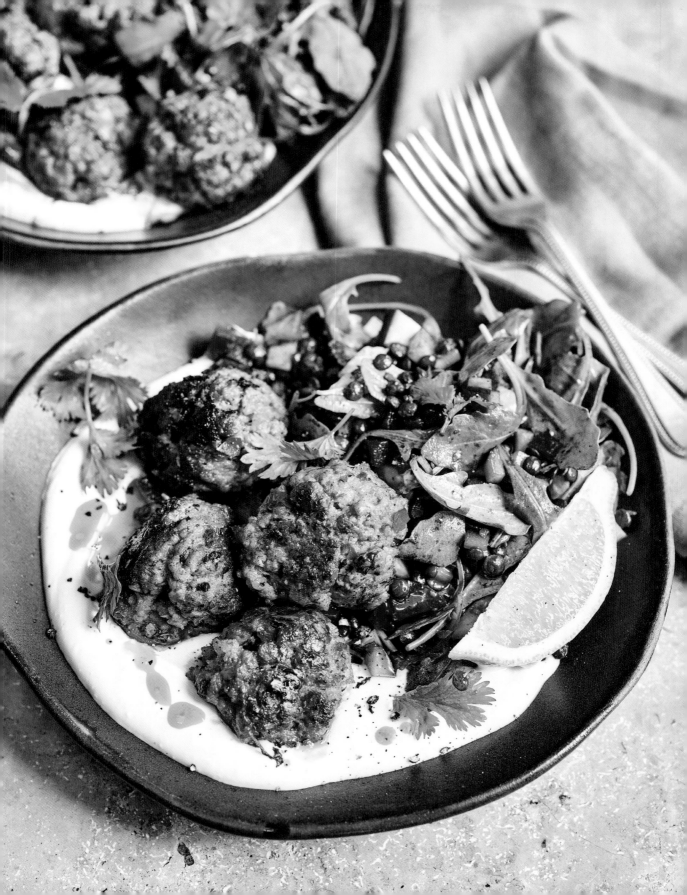

SAUCY SPRING ONION CHICKEN

This is one of my family's favourite recipes, and it went down a storm when I shared it on Instagram. Everyone loved it. It takes spring onions and makes them the star of the dish, which creates so much flavour. It's halfway between a stir-fry and a curry, with a lovely thick sauce that coats the whole lot and will have you licking the plate clean.

SERVES 4

1 tbsp vegetable oil
640g (1lb 6oz) chicken
  mini fillets
40g (1½oz) cornflour
5 tbsp oyster sauce
4 tbsp soy sauce
2 tbsp honey
2 bunches of spring onions,
  finely sliced
4 garlic cloves, grated
thumb-sized piece of fresh
  ginger, peeled and grated
200–400ml (7–14fl oz)
  water
juice of 1–2 limes, plus
  wedges to serve

1 Heat the oil in a large frying pan or wok and fry the chicken over a high heat for 3–4 minutes, so it gets some nice golden colour.

2 While the chicken is browning, whisk together the cornflour, oyster sauce, soy sauce and honey in a small bowl. Set aside.

3 Scatter in most of the spring onions, setting aside some to garnish, along with the garlic and ginger and stir-fry for 1 minute until fragrant.

4 Pour in the cornflour-soy mixture and coat the chicken and veg, then add the water, bring up to the boil and let the whole thing bubble away and get thick and glossy.

5 Season with lime juice, to taste. Serve with rice and lime wedges and scatter with the remaining spring onions.

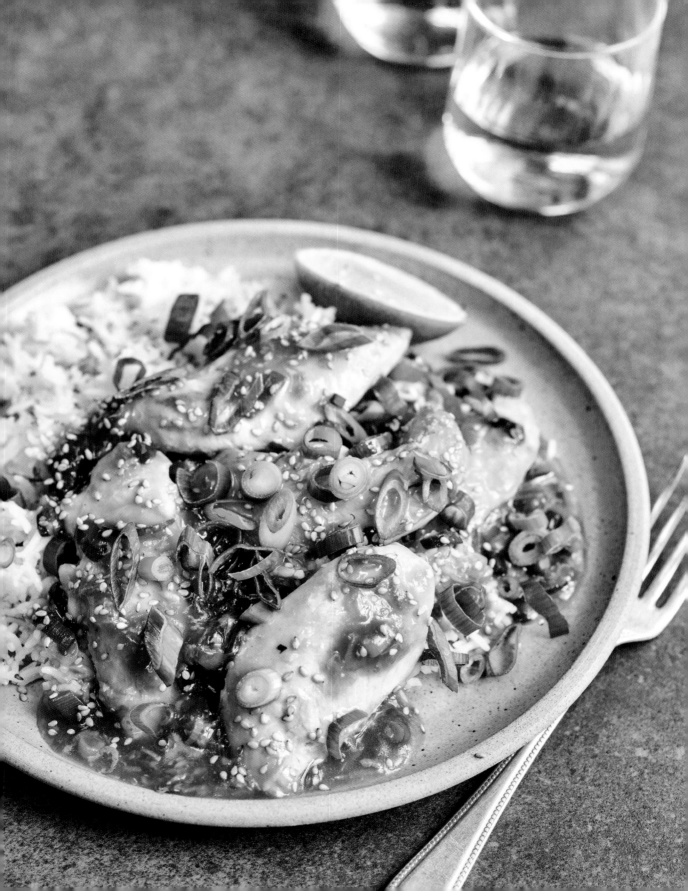

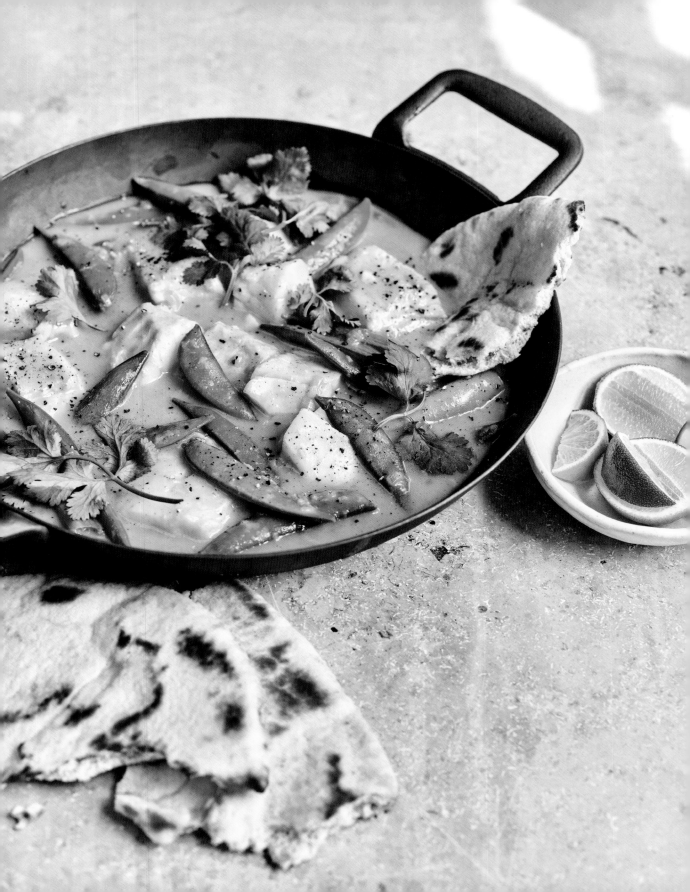

COCONUT CURRY COD

I'll be honest with you. I don't like things that have a very fishy taste and would usually choose a chicken curry over a fish curry, but this one using cod is absolutely delicious. It's mild and fragrant and one I love to eat with the kids. Serve with rice or mop up all the sauce with warm flatbreads.

SERVES 4

1 tbsp vegetable oil
1 banana shallot, finely chopped
3 garlic cloves, grated
thumb-sized piece of fresh ginger, peeled and grated
1 lemongrass stick, bashed
1 tbsp garam masala
1 tsp ground turmeric
400ml (14oz) tin of coconut milk
200ml (7fl oz) vegetable stock
200g (7oz) sugar snap peas
400g (14oz) skinless cod fillets, cut into chunks
1 tsp maple syrup (optional)
juice of 1 lime
handful of fresh coriander leaves, to garnish
rice or flatbreads, to serve

1 Heat the oil in a deep frying pan and fry the shallot, garlic and ginger and drop in the whole lemongrass stick until it smells fragrant and is beginning to soften, around 3 minutes.

2 Add the garam masala and turmeric with a tiny splash of water and cook for 1 minute.

3 Pour in the coconut milk and vegetable stock, then bring to a boil. Add the sugar snaps and cook for 2 minutes, then add the cod. Space out the chunks evenly, toss to coat, then cook for 3–4 minutes on a low heat with a lid on until the fish is opaque and cooked through. Season the curry to taste with a decent amount of salt, lots of fresh lime juice and if it needs it, a little dash of maple syrup to balance it.

4 Serve with a handful of coriander leaves and rice or flatbreads.

STICKY PORK BELLY + KIMCHI FRIED RICE

I don't often cook pork belly at home, but I always order it when I eat out because I love it and when it's cooked well it tastes outrageous. Covered in this miso honey glaze, it gets seriously sweet and sticky – it's completely moreish. And it's a match made in heaven with the tangy, spicy kimchi fried rice.

SERVES 2

250g (9oz) pork belly
  strips, cut into cubes
1½ tbsp miso paste
4 tbsp soy sauce
2 tbsp vegetable oil
1 tbsp honey
1 large pak choi, cut into
  quarters
200g (7oz) kimchi
250g (9oz) pouch of
  microwaveable rice
2 eggs

To serve (optional)
2 spring onions, finely
  chopped
1 tbsp toasted sesame
  seeds

1 Add the pork to a bowl with the miso paste, 2 tablespoons of the soy sauce and 1 tablespoon of the vegetable oil. Mix until combined.

2 Heat a frying pan and add the pork, cook over a medium–high heat for 7–10 minutes, then drizzle over the honey for the final minute of cooking until the pork is golden and cooked through. Remove the pork from the pan and set aside on a plate. Add in the pak choi with a splash of water and cook until tender.

3 Heat the remaining oil in another frying pan. Add the kimchi, rice and the remaining soy sauce. Fry for 30 seconds over a high heat before pushing the rice mix to one side, adding the eggs and vigorously stirring the eggs while frying until they look scrambled. Mix this through with the rest of the kimchi rice.

4 Serve the pork and pak choi over the rice with any remaining juices. Sprinkle over the spring onion and sesame seeds.

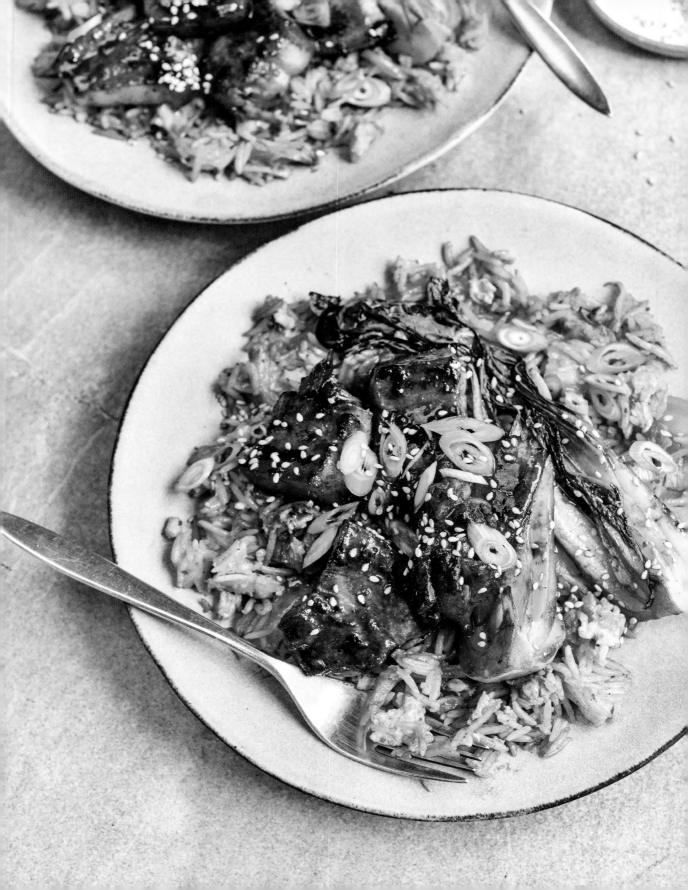

CHICKEN FAJITA PIE

OK, so, this isn't technically a 15-minute meal, as you need to bake it for 15 minutes, but I have a filo pie in every single book I've ever written, so I just had to include one. It's a tradition! I thought I had run out of ideas, but then it hit me: chicken fajita is one of the best flavours ever, so why not try it in a pie? The result is incredible.

SERVES 4

3 skinless, boneless chicken breasts, sliced into strips
3 peppers, deseeded and sliced into strips
1 large red onion, sliced
150g (5oz) cherry tomatoes (leave whole)
1½ tsp chipotle paste
1 tsp smoked paprika
2 tbsp olive oil, plus extra to drizzle
pinch of salt
100g (3½oz) Cheddar cheese, grated
½ pack of filo pastry
small handful of fresh coriander leaves, to garnish

1 Preheat the oven to 200°C, 180°C fan, gas mark 6.

2 Add the chicken, peppers, onion, tomatoes, chipotle paste, paprika and olive oil to a bowl with a pinch of salt. Toss to combine and coat.

3 Heat a large ovenproof frying pan, and fry off the chicken and veg until the veg has softened and the chicken has a golden tinge, around 6–7 minutes – don't worry about it being fully cooked through.

4 Sprinkle the Cheddar on top of the chicken and pepper mixture, then scrunch filo sheets on top to totally cover. Drizzle with a little bit of olive oil, if you like, then transfer the pan into the oven and bake for 12–15 minutes until the pastry is golden and crisp.

5 Sprinkle over the coriander leaves and enjoy.

TIP/SWAP

Make this into more of a feast by serving with soured cream, avocado slices, a cabbage slaw or a nice bit of salad.

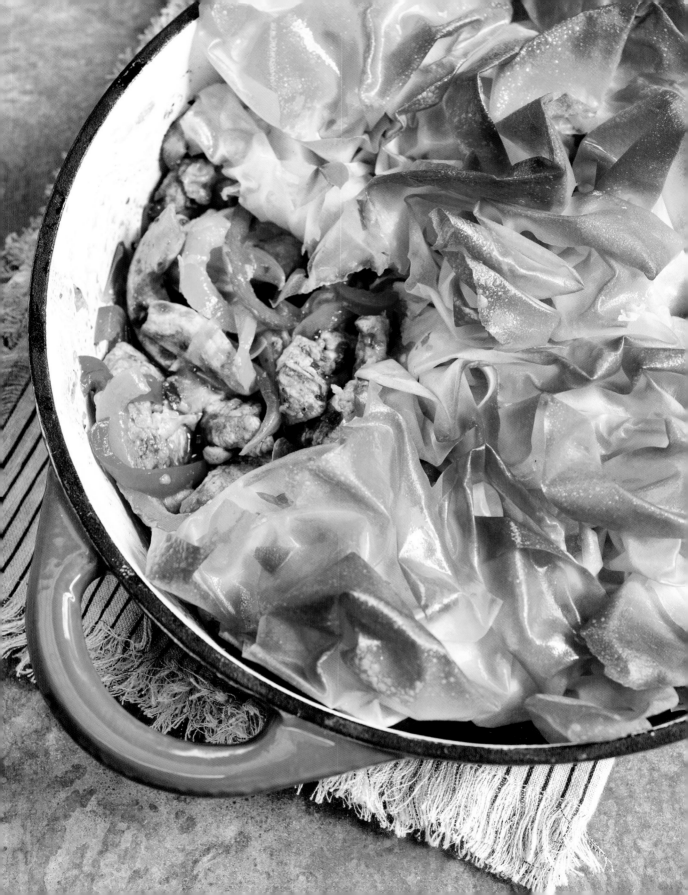

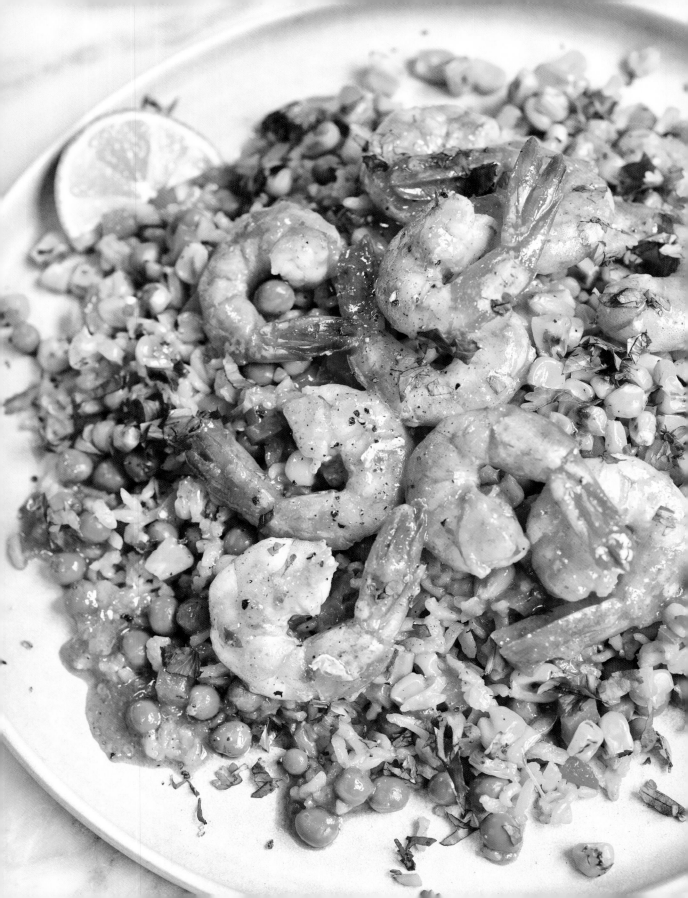

PERI-PERI PRAWNS WITH CHARRED CORN + SPICY RICE

I love, love, love this recipe. It's packed full of flavour and uses some of my favourite herbs and spices. I like having this at home or also on the go for lunch. If you're not a fan of prawns, make this with sliced chicken breast instead.

SERVES 2

200g (7oz) tin of sweetcorn, drained
250g (9oz) pouch of cooked brown rice
½ tsp ground turmeric
½ tsp smoked paprika
¼ tsp chilli flakes (optional)
100g (3½oz) frozen peas
½ red pepper, deseeded and finely diced
small handful of fresh coriander, finely chopped
zest and juice of 1 lime
200g (7oz) raw king prawns
oil, for frying (optional)
4 tbsp peri-peri sauce
salt and freshly ground black pepper

1 Add the sweetcorn to a dry frying pan and cook over a high heat until charred – around 5 minutes.

2 In the meantime, tip out the rice pouch into a microwave-safe dish and add the turmeric, smoked paprika, chilli flakes, if using, frozen peas and red pepper. Stir well to combine, then pour over 60ml (2½fl oz) water, cover with cling film, and microwave for 3 minutes until fragrant and fluffy. Mix well with a fork and set aside.

3 Once the corn has charred, remove from the pan and season with salt, pepper, coriander and the lime zest and juice. Set aside.

4 Toss the prawns into the pan you used for the corn, with a tiny splash of oil if needed and fry for 1 minute on each side until fully pink through. Pour in the peri-peri sauce and let it bubble up – use a wooden spoon to scrape up any flavour from the bottom of the pan, then serve with the rice and corn.

'NDUJA CARBONARA

I'm about to make a big statement: I think this is one of the top five tastiest recipes in the book. You really don't want to skip this one. 'Nduja is a spicy Italian chilli paste made with pork – it's rich, fiery and completely delicious. You can find it in jars in most supermarkets, or in a deli as a fresh slab – either are totally fine. This will not disappoint.

SERVES 4

350g (12oz) spaghetti or bucatini
150g (5oz) pancetta cubes
4 tbsp 'nduja paste
4 egg yolks, plus 2 eggs
75g (3oz) Parmesan, finely grated, plus extra to serve
salt and freshly ground black pepper

1 Get the kettle on, then pour the boiling water into a large pot and salt generously. Boil the pasta for 9–10 minutes until al dente.

2 Pop the pancetta into a large frying pan and dry-fry over a low heat until crispy and the fat has rendered. Add the 'nduja paste, stir for 1 minute until fragrant, then turn off the heat.

3 Mix together the egg yolks, whole eggs and Parmesan in a large bowl with lots of black pepper.

4 When the pasta is al dente, use a slotted spoon or tongs to transfer it directly into the pancetta and 'nduja pan. Turn the heat to low and mix well to combine.

5 Turn off the heat again and pour in the egg and Parmesan mixture and toss well off the heat until the sauce is glossy and clings to the pasta – you may need to use a mugful or two of pasta water to get it there, tossing vigorously all the while.

6 Serve up with a bit of extra Parmesan and enjoy.

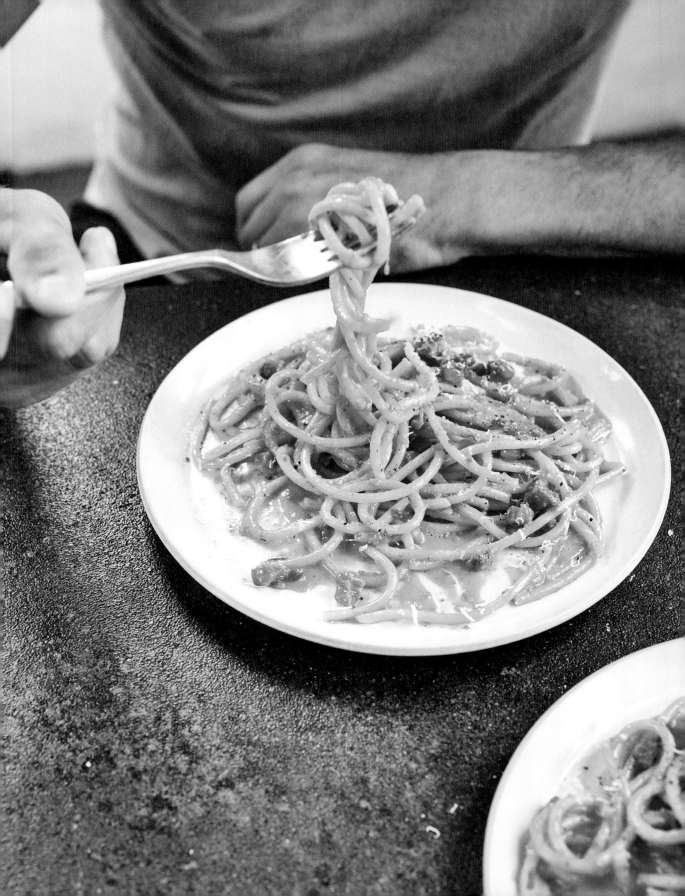

CAESAR SCHNITZEL

I love the flavour of Chicken Caesar so much I decided to put my own spin on it here. The yoghurty Caesar-style dressing is ready in a heartbeat. I've left out the anchovies, but do add a couple if you like. There are a few things going on at once to get this on the table in 15 minutes, but it's worth it.

SERVES 2

350g (12oz) baby potatoes
8 slices of thin pancetta
2 skinless, boneless
  chicken breasts
4 tbsp plain flour
1 egg
40g (1½oz) dried
  breadcrumbs
vegetable oil, for frying
200g (7oz) green beans
100g (3½oz) natural
  yoghurt
1 garlic clove
50g (2oz) Parmesan,
  grated, plus extra to serve
10g (¼oz) capers
1 tsp Dijon mustard
juice of ½ lemon, plus extra
  to serve
2 tbsp red wine vinegar
1 tbsp extra-virgin olive oil
½ bunch of fresh chives,
  finely chopped
salt and freshly ground
  black pepper

1 Pop the kettle on. Once boiling, get the potatoes in a large saucepan, cover with the boiling water and set over a high heat. Set a timer for 8 minutes.

2 Meanwhile, preheat your grill to its highest setting and lay the pancetta slices on a baking tray. Grill for 2 minutes until crisp. Set aside.

3 Use a knife to cut a slit into the thickest part of the chicken breast to open it out. Season with salt, then lay in between two pieces of non-stick baking paper or cling film and bash with a rolling pin or the base of a frying pan to flatten. Sprinkle 2 tablespoons of the flour over each chicken breast directly on the baking paper to coat thoroughly.

4 Crack the egg into a shallow bowl and whisk with a fork, and pop the breadcrumbs into another bowl. Coat the chicken in the egg, then the breadcrumbs.

5 Add enough vegetable oil to a frying pan to coat the base of the pan and heat over a medium heat.

6 By now, your 8-minute timer should be up, so add the green beans to the potatoes and set a timer for 4 more minutes.

7 Fry the chicken breasts in the oil for 2–3 minutes on each side until deeply golden and cooked through.

8 Blitz together the yoghurt, garlic, Parmesan, capers, Dijon mustard and lemon juice. Season to taste.

9 Drain the potatoes and green beans. Roughly break apart the potatoes with a fork, add the red wine vinegar, oil, chives and tear in the pancetta. Season generously.

10 Serve the chicken with the green bean potatoes, a big dollop of the yoghurt dressing and a squeeze of lemon.

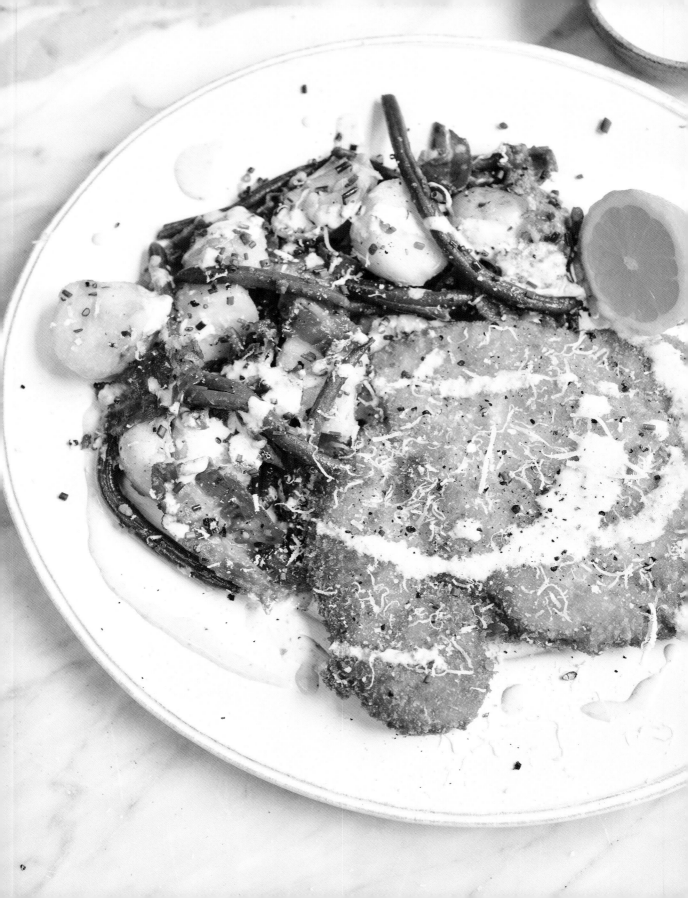

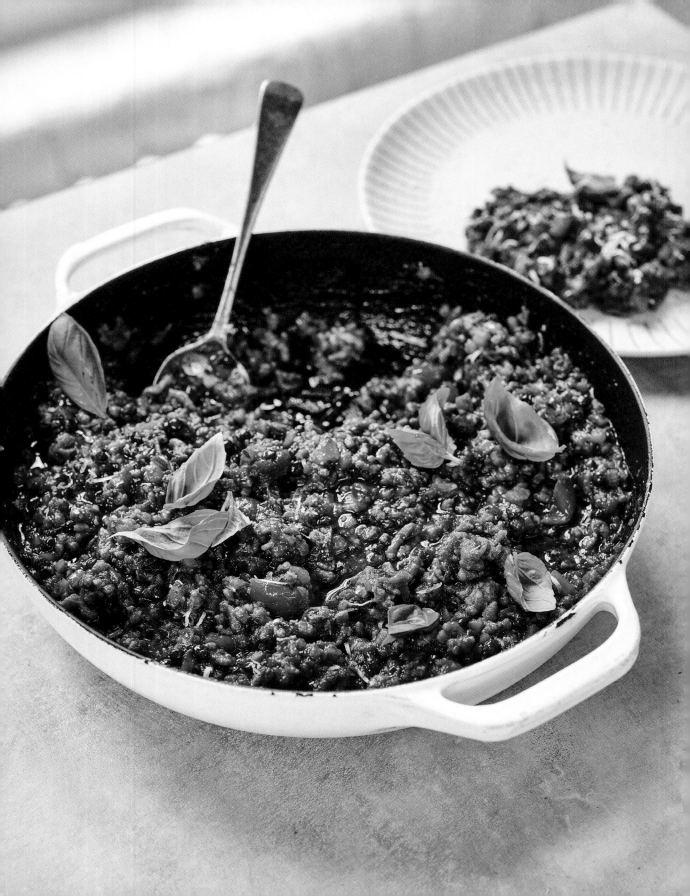

LAMB MINCE RAGU

This tastes as good as it looks. A food processor is your friend here; quickly blitzing the celery, carrot and onions means that you don't waste time chopping and can get a lip-smacking ragu in minutes. Lamb mince is super soft and doesn't require the slow cooking that you would expect from a ragu – and we've added a big blob of Marmite to give it that slow-cooked meaty taste. I've paired it here with a wild rice pouch, but go for any grains, quick polenta or spaghetti depending on what you love.

SERVES 4

2 carrots
1 celery stick
1 onion
2 tbsp olive oil
2 tsp dried oregano
500g (1lb 2oz) lamb mince
250g (9oz) pouch of puy lentils
1 tbsp yeast extract (we like Marmite)
1 jar of sun-dried tomatoes, drained
400ml (14fl oz) passata
1 tbsp balsamic vinegar
salt and freshly ground black pepper

To serve
grated Parmesan
large handful of fresh basil leaves

1 Cut the carrots, celery and onion into manageable chunks and pulse in the food processor until it looks finely chopped – don't let it turn into soup.

2 Heat the olive oil in a large saucepan or casserole dish over medium heat, then follow with the carrot, celery and onion mixture and dried oregano and cook for 4 minutes until it's softened and the moisture has evaporated. Add the lamb mince and break up well with the back of a wooden spoon. Once the lamb is cooked through (after around 8 minutes), add the lentils, Marmite, sun-dried tomatoes and passata and cook over a high heat for 2–3 minutes or until the tomato has reduced slightly and been absorbed by the meat.

3 Season generously with salt, pepper and vinegar.

4 Serve spooned over your grain pouch with lots of grated Parmesan and fresh basil.

TIP/SWAP

You can find fresh or frozen 'sofrito' often in your supermarket – it's a pre-chopped version of the celery, carrot and onion mix, which will save you even more time.

SPEEDY SMASH BURGERS

Oh my word. Just look at that burger. It's a masterpiece. I personally believe there is nothing more satisfying in life than a good burger. This one isn't just good, though; it's out of this world. It's the ultimate Californian, West Coast burger. A true classic that you will want to make over and over again.

MAKES 3 BURGERS

3 burger buns, split
2 onions, thinly sliced
1 tsp vegetable oil
500g (1lb 2oz) beef mince
3 tbsp yellow mustard
6 slices of cheese
½ iceberg lettuce,
   shredded
salt and freshly ground
   black pepper

Burger sauce
3 tbsp mayonnaise
2 tbsp ketchup
2 tbsp yellow mustard
6 pickled jalapeños, finely
   chopped

TIP/SWAP
Swap the pickled jalapenos for a gherkin if you want a more traditional flavour.

1 Heat 2 large frying pans – to get this done in 15 minutes you're going to need to divide and conquer!

2 In one pan, toast the burger buns cut side down in the dry pan until toasted and slightly charred.

3 In the other pan, throw in the onions with the oil and cook over a high heat until slightly softened and starting to char around the edges.

4 In the meantime, mix together all the ingredients for the burger sauce. Set aside. Divide the mince into 6 even balls.

5 Remove the burger buns and onions from the pans. Working one burger ball at a time, turn the heat right up (and get the extractor fan on!), then place a burger patty into the dry pan and press down with a burger press or a heavy based saucepan really, really hard until the burger smashes down completely flat. You'll need to space the burger patties far enough away from each other to allow this to happen. Repeat with all the burger patties, then season with salt, pepper and ½ teaspoon yellow mustard on each uncooked side of beef.

6 Cook for 2 minutes on the first side until deeply golden and getting crispy, then flip and add a cheese slice to the cooked side of each burger. Cook for a further 1–2 minutes until the cheese has melted and the burger edges are nicely caramelised.

7 Load up the buns with sauce on the bottom, followed by lettuce, two patties and then even more sauce.

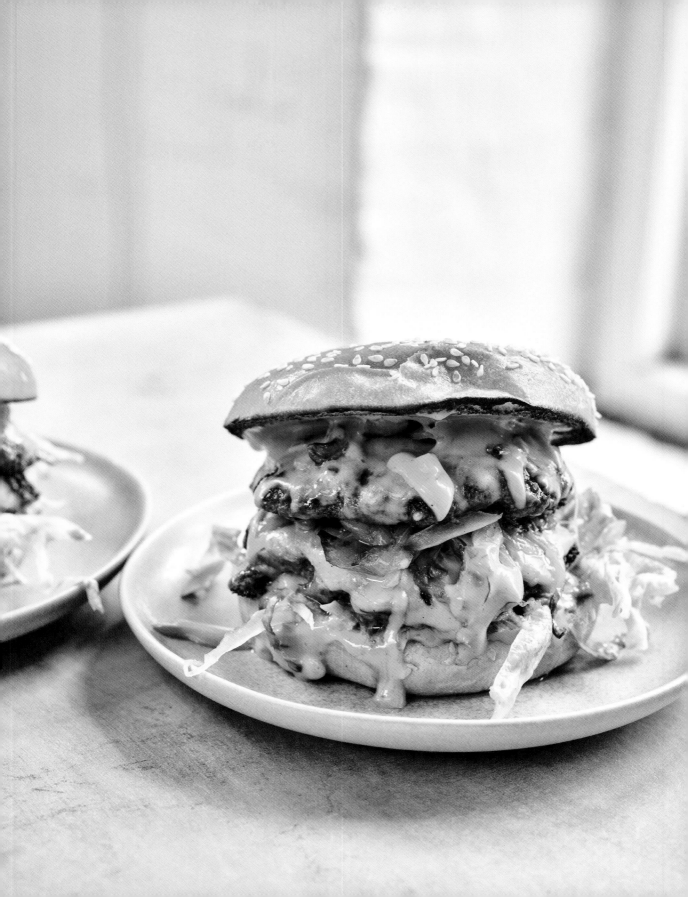

SESAME CHICKEN THIGHS WITH SPICY SATAY SLAW

This is one of mine and Rosie's absolute favourites – we love a satay, and we love spicy food even more, and using chilli oil in the sauce really gives it a kick. This is perfect to make on the barbecue, too.

SERVES 2

1 tbsp sesame oil
4–6 skinless, boneless
  chicken thighs (quantity
  depends on size)
3 tbsp sesame seeds
3 tbsp soy sauce
1 tbsp honey
100g (3½oz) sugar snaps,
  cut in half
¼ red cabbage, shredded
2 carrots, julienned (or very
  thinly sliced into batons)
½ cucumber, julienned
  (or very thinly sliced into
  batons)
handful of fresh mint leaves
handful of fresh coriander
  leaves

Slaw dressing

4 tbsp peanut butter
3 tbsp soy sauce
2 tsp chilli oil
juice of 1 lime, plus extra
  wedges to serve
1 lemongrass stick, finely
  chopped
thumb-sized piece of fresh
  ginger, peeled and finely
  chopped

1 Heat the sesame oil in a large frying pan, then add the chicken thighs. Cook for 4–5 minutes until golden and cooked through, then add the sesame seeds, soy sauce and honey and cook until sticky and coated, another 2–3 minutes.

2 In the meantime, mix together the dressing for the spicy satay slaw.

3 Toss together the sugar snaps, cabbage, carrots, cucumber and herbs and drizzle over the dressing.

4 Plate up the chicken thighs with a lime wedge and plenty of spicy slaw.

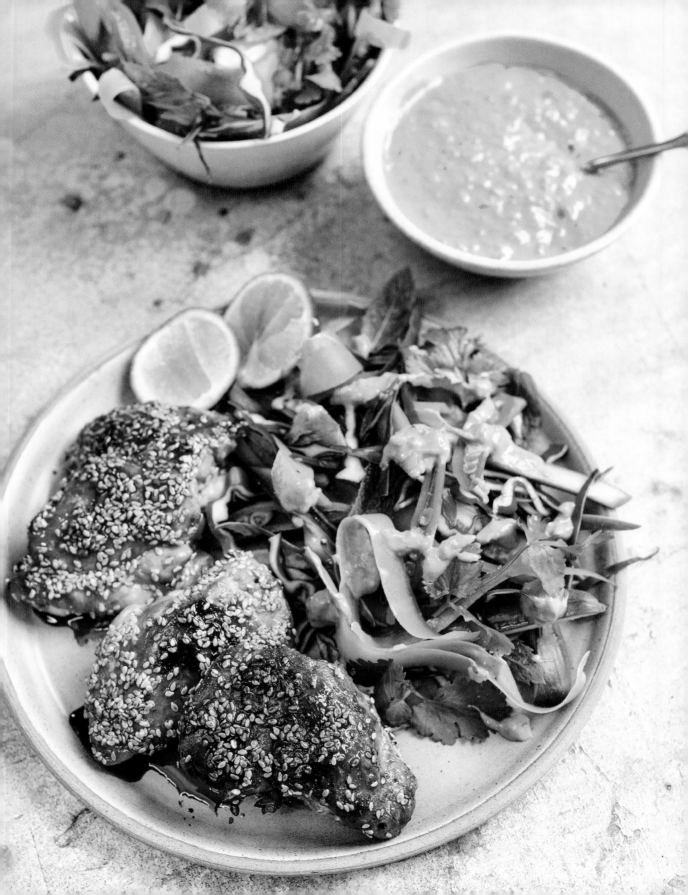

TOMATO CHICKEN CURRY

This delicious chicken curry is a quicker, healthier, cheat's version of a chicken makhani and you won't believe how good it tastes in so little time. It's a great one to have in your back pocket when people are hungry and you need to get dinner on the table, quick! Serve with rice, naan or chapatis.

SERVES 4

1 tbsp vegetable oil
1 onion, finely chopped
3 garlic cloves, finely chopped
thumb-sized piece of ginger, peeled and finely chopped
3 tbsp mild curry paste
2 tbsp tomato purée
6 boneless chicken thighs, cut into cubes
400ml (14fl oz) tin of coconut milk
250g (9oz) tomatoes, cut into chunks
200g (7oz) spinach leaves
juice of 1 lime
salt and freshly ground black pepper

To serve
handful of fresh coriander (optional)
rice, naan or chapatis

1 Add the oil to a frying pan with the onion, garlic and ginger and cook over a medium heat for 2–3 minutes to begin to soften. Add the curry paste and tomato purée and cook for 2 minutes until fragrant and beginning to separate.

2 Add the chicken, coconut milk and tomatoes and cook for 10–12 minutes until the chicken is cooked through. Add in the spinach and stir until wilted.

3 Season to taste generously with salt and pepper and add lime juice. Serve with coriander and sides of your choice.

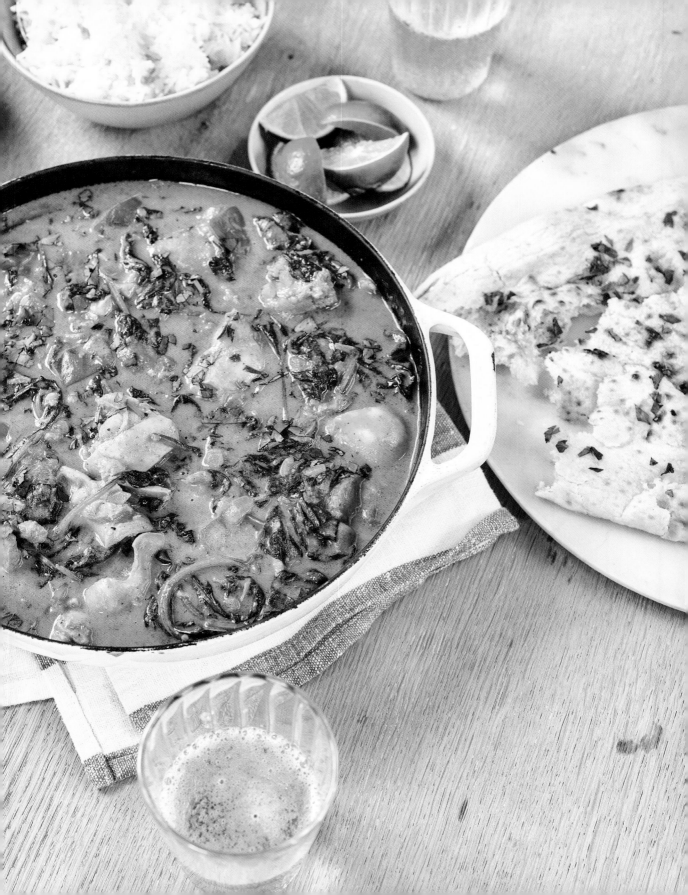

SNACKS + DESSERTS

This chapter includes some delicious but really simple snacks to help with that mid-afternoon struggle, as well as some healthy treats to satisfy any cravings.

For those of you (like me) who like a little treat now and then, but don't want the energy slump once you've eaten them, I've included a few healthy spins on desserts, which are packed with fresh fruits and less sugar – you can even change some of them up to make the most of what's in season or to use your favourite fruits. This is about ditching the guilt and allowing you to whip up a little treat that makes you and your body feel good.

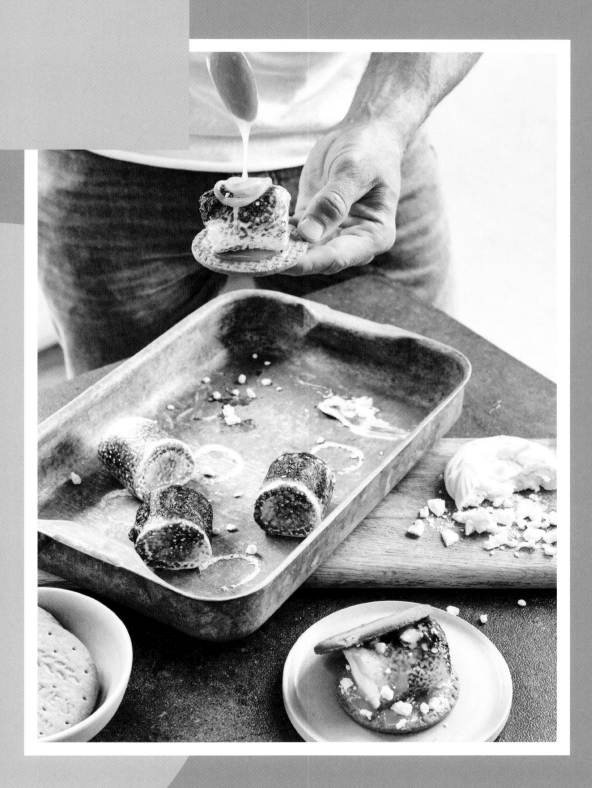

CHEESE, AVOCADO + MARMITE CRUMPETS

V

You can't beat a good crumpet, and this little afternoon treat is a combination made in heaven. You're going to have to trust me on this one; the combination of salty Marmite, hot cheese and cold avocado is a winner.

SERVES 2

2 crumpets
30g (1oz) Cheddar cheese, grated
½ large avocado, sliced
1 tbsp Marmite
seeds of your choice, to serve

1 Preheat the grill to its highest setting.

2 Pop the crumpets in the toaster for 1½ minutes. Spread with Marmite and sprinkle over the grated cheese, then grill until melted, around 1–2 minutes.

3 Top with sliced avocado and seeds and enjoy.

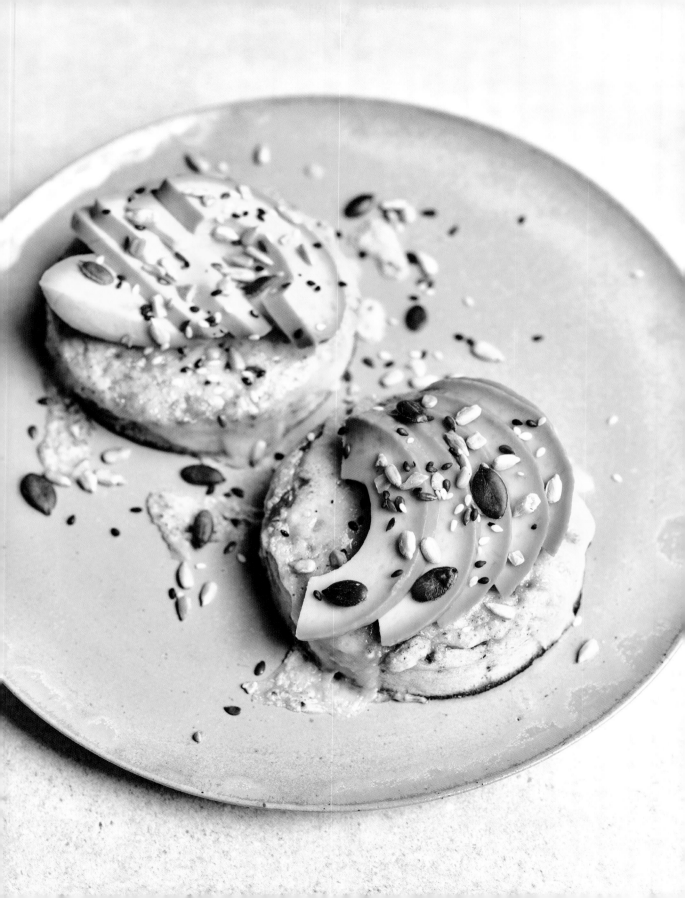

LIME PICKLE FROZEN VEG FRITTERS

VG

If you've got a vegetable, you can fritter it. These pakora style fritters are a brilliant way of using up frozen veg and making it ten times more delicious. The lime pickle adds that extra something and helps to make these completely moreish.

MAKES 10 SMALL FRITTERS

75g (3oz) gram flour
5 tbsp water
150g (5oz) frozen mixed
  vegetables
2 tbsp lime pickle, roughly
  chopped
1 green chilli, finely
  chopped
small bunch of fresh
  coriander, finely
  chopped, plus extra to
  garnish
2–3 tbsp vegetable oil
dairy-free yoghurt, to serve
  (optional)

1 In a bowl, whisk together the gram flour and water until you have a paste. Toss through the vegetables, lime pickle, green chilli and chopped coriander – it won't be like a batter, but everything should be coated by the gram flour mixture.

2 Pour the oil into a frying pan until it coats the base of the pan – you're looking to shallow-fry these to make sure they're nice and crispy.

3 When the oil shimmers, fry heaped tablespoons of the mixture for each fritter, turning to cook and get golden on each side, around 4 minutes total.

4 Serve with extra coriander and a dollop of dairy-free yoghurt, if you like.

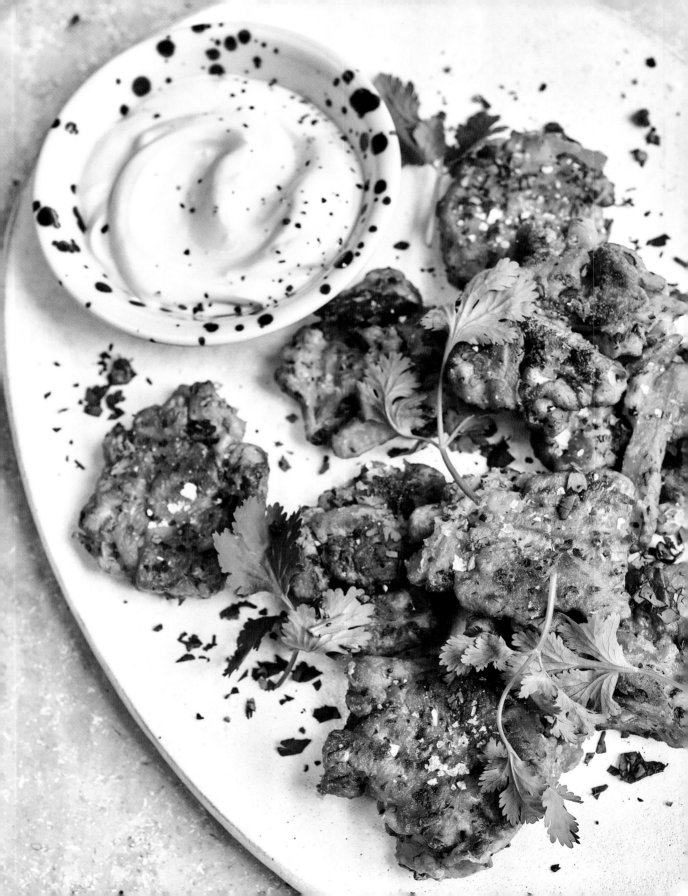

CRISPY PARMESAN ARTICHOKES

V

I love to keep a tin of artichoke hearts in the cupboard for when the craving hits – they're loaded with nutrients and are completely delicious. Feel free to leave the chilli out of the marinara sauce if that's not your thing. These definitely come out the crispiest from the air fryer, but they're still very good from the oven.

SERVES 2–4 AS A SNACK

20g (¾oz) panko breadcrumbs
15g (½oz) Parmesan, grated, plus extra to serve
400g (14oz) tin of artichoke hearts, drained and cut in half
oil spray
2 tbsp extra-virgin olive oil
4 garlic cloves, grated
1 red chilli, finely chopped
400ml (14fl oz) passata
1 tbsp red wine vinegar
small handful of fresh flat-leaf parsley, finely chopped
salt and freshly ground black pepper

1 If using an oven, preheat to 200°C, 180°C fan, gas mark 6.

2 Mix together the breadcrumbs and the Parmesan in a shallow bowl.

3 Spray the artichoke halves with oil spray, dunk them into the breadcrumb mixture on all sides, then place them on a baking tray lined with non-stick baking paper.

4 Spray again with oil, then bake for 12–14 minutes until golden and crisp. Alternatively, add to your air fryer basket and air-fry at 200°C for 12 minutes until golden and crisp.

5 While the artichokes are roasting, add the olive oil to a medium saucepan and heat on a medium–high heat. Add the garlic and chilli and fry for 1–2 minutes until fragrant and sizzling. Pour in the passata, turn the heat down and simmer for the duration that the artichokes remain in the oven. Then season generously with salt and pepper and add red wine vinegar, to taste.

6 Serve the crispy artichokes with the marinara sauce and a sprinkling of parsley and extra Parmesan.

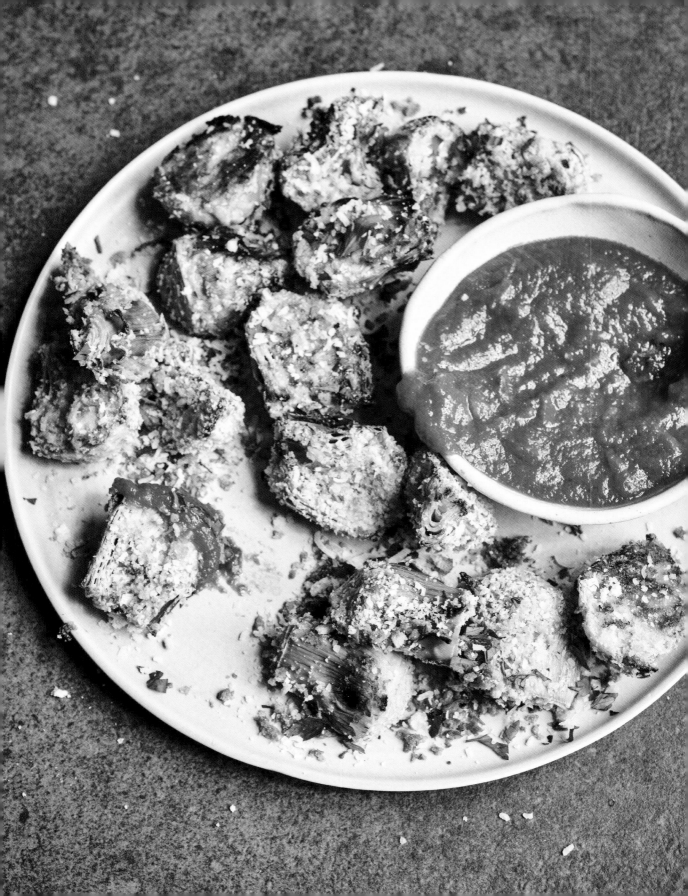

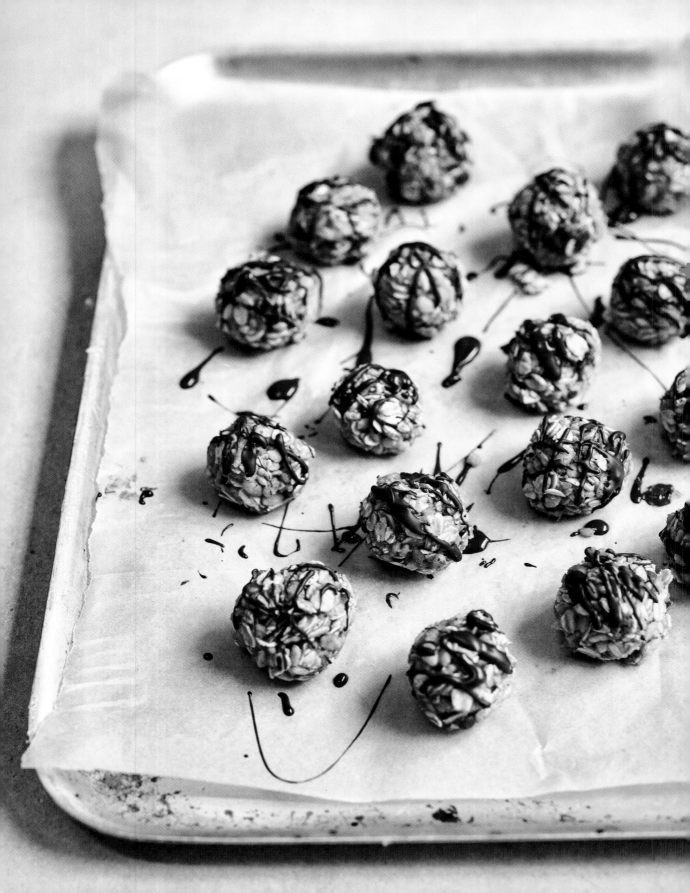

RICE POP ENERGY BITES

These little balls of goodness are perfect for an afternoon pick-me-up, and if you have little ones they're also great for weaning, as they have no added sugar and are both crunchy and portable. Beware, as they are very moreish and you may end up eating the whole batch by yourself.

MAKES 12 BALLS

1 large banana, peeled (about 100g/3½oz)
50g (2oz) peanut butter
6 tbsp oats
20g (¾oz) mixed seeds
40g (1½oz) rice pops or crisp breakfast cereal
50g dark chocolate, melted (optional)

1 In a bowl, mash the banana well and combine with the peanut butter until smooth.

2 Stir through the oats, seeds and the rice pops.

3 Form into 12 golf-ball-sized bites, drizzle with chocolate (if using) and refrigerate until you're ready to eat them – they will keep in the fridge for up to 4 days.

STOVETOP PLUM CRUMBLE *PLUMBLE*

VG

A crumble with no faffing about. Can you believe it? No faff, no oven and it's ready in 15 minutes! This speedy crumble has a few healthy shortcuts, but the end result is bang on. Tastes just as good when it hits the lips. Swap the plums for any in-season fruit and follow the same method – you may just need to lengthen the cooking times for harder fruits like apples and pears.

SERVES 2

300g (10oz) plums
 (approx. 4), stones
 removed
1 tbsp, plus 20g (¾oz)
 demerara sugar
½ tsp vanilla extract
30g (1oz) salted butter
30g (1oz) hazelnuts,
 roughly chopped
40g (1½oz) porridge oats
20g (¾oz) plain flour
1 tsp ground cinnamon

1 Add the plums, the 1 tablespoon of sugar and vanilla extract to a small saucepan with 2 tablespoons of water. Cook over a high heat with the lid on for 5 minutes, then take off the lid and reduce the heat, cooking for a further 2–3 minutes, until the fruit is soft.

2 In a frying pan, add the remaining demerara sugar, butter, hazelnuts, oats, flour and cinnamon and cook, stirring regularly, until golden and crisp, about 10 minutes.

3 Divide the fruit between two bowls and sprinkle with the crumble mixture to serve.

→ **TIP/SWAP**
Add any nuts, seeds or even granola to the crumble to mix it up.

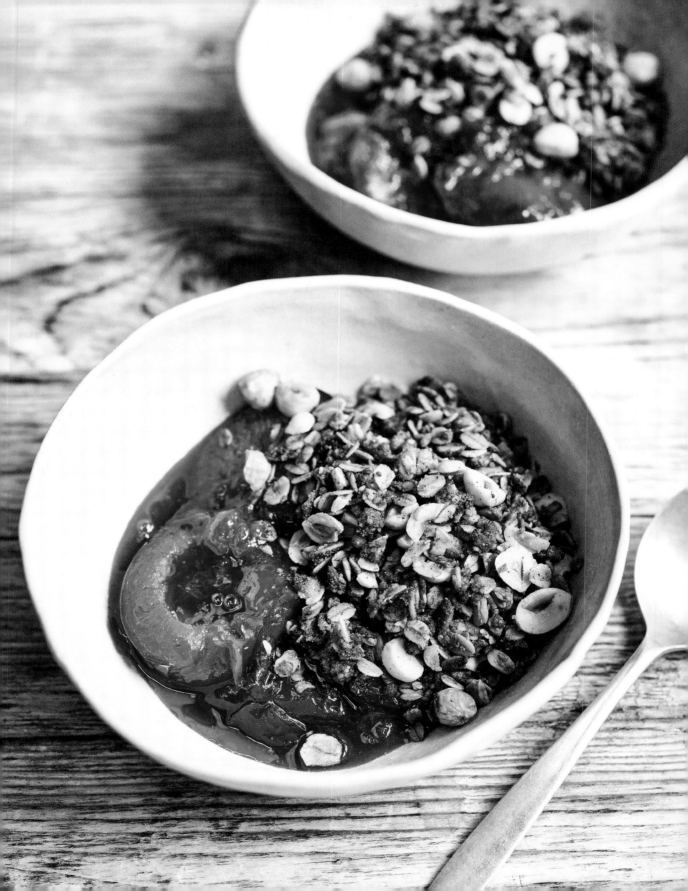

STEAMED MARMALADE PUDDING

VG

If you know me, you know I love marmalade. I'm literally worse than Paddington Bear. I've got a whole shelf in my fridge dedicated to my marmalade collection. So I thought it was only right to create a pudding using my favourite ingredient. This nostalgic pud is vegan and is made in the microwave, so it's the fastest, most impressive pudding you'll make this year. Swap the marmalade for golden syrup or jam if you're not as much of a fan.

SERVES 4

margarine or oil spray, to grease
5 tbsp marmalade
75g (3oz) caster sugar
75g (3oz) vegetable oil
150g (5oz) self-raising flour
125ml (4fl oz) dairy-free milk (I like to use soya)
½ tbsp apple cider vinegar
1 tsp baking powder
a pinch of salt

1 Grease a large microwave-safe pudding bowl. Spoon the marmalade into the base and set aside.

2 In a separate mixing bowl, mix together all of the rest of the ingredients until smooth.

3 Pour the mixture into the pudding bowl, cover with cling film, then cook for 2–3 minutes on high until the mixture is risen, puffy and there are no visible bits of wet batter.

4 Run a knife around the edge of the cake, then tip out onto a plate and eat immediately.

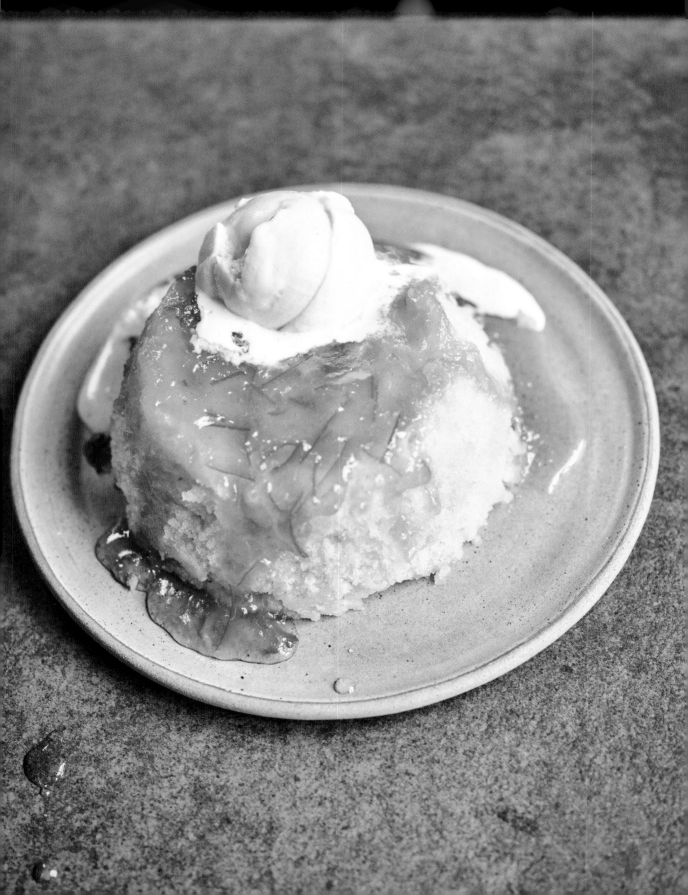

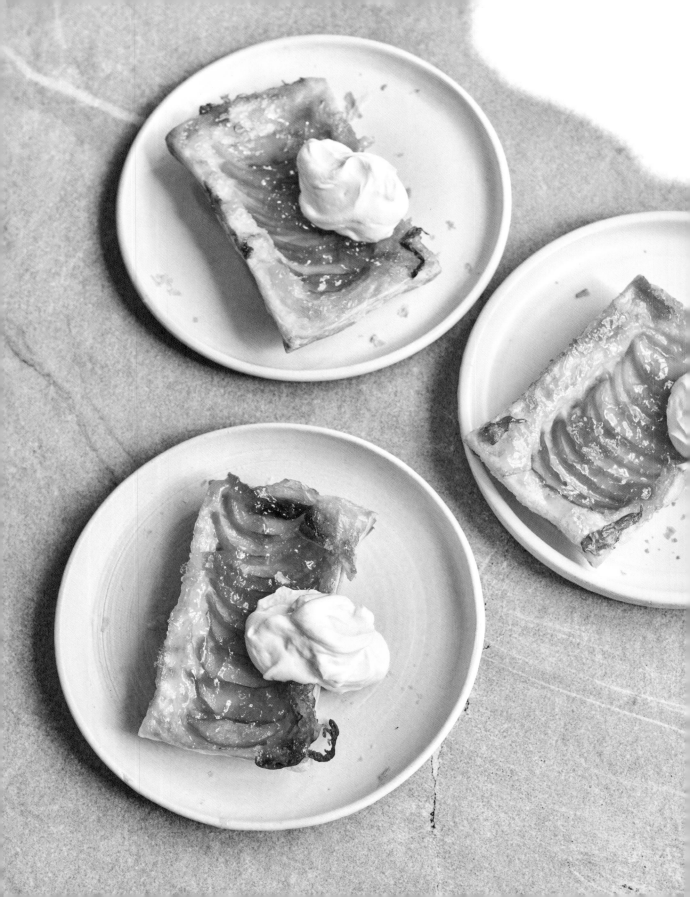

APRICOT + APPLE TARTLETS

These tasty tartlets use the hack of baking individual puff pastries upside down – it helps the fruit to caramelise quicker, and allows the pastry to get lovely and golden brown without going soggy. A win-win.

MAKES 8

1 sheet of ready-to-roll
  puff pastry
2 tsp apricot jam
3 apples, thinly sliced
1 egg, beaten
vanilla ice cream, to serve

1 Preheat the oven to 200°C, 180°C fan, gas mark 6.

2 Roll out the puff pastry and cut in half lengthways, then into 4 sections vertically, leaving you with 8 rectangles.

3 Spoon the apricot jam directly into one section of the baking tray, then arrange 4–5 slices of apple on top of the jam in a rectangular pattern – bear in mind that these will need to be completely covered by the pastry, so keep it packed in tight. Cover the apples with the pastry, using cupped hands to push down around the fruit to make it secure and use a fork to crimp down at the edges. Coat with egg wash and repeat with the remaining rectangles.

4 Bake for 10–12 minutes until golden and puffy. Serve each tartlet with a scoop of vanilla ice cream.

MICROWAVE GINGER MUG CAKE

v

There's nothing better than having a craving for cake and realising you can make one in 2 minutes flat. Spiced, fluffy and sweet, this mug cake really hits the spot – especially with a scoop of vanilla ice cream!

MAKES 1

1 tbsp butter
2 tbsp black treacle
2 tbsp whole milk
1 tsp vanilla extract
5 tbsp plain flour
¼ tsp baking powder
¼ tsp ground ginger
½ tsp mixed spice
ice cream, to serve
  (optional)

1 Put the butter into a mug and microwave for 15–20 seconds until melted.

2 Swirl the butter around the inside of the mug, then add the treacle, milk and vanilla. Mix well to combine. Add the flour, baking powder and spices and mix again to ensure everything is thoroughly combined.

3 Microwave for 1 minute 15 seconds–1 minute 30 seconds, depending on your microwave, until the cakes have risen and cooked through.

4 Eat immediately with ice cream, if you like.

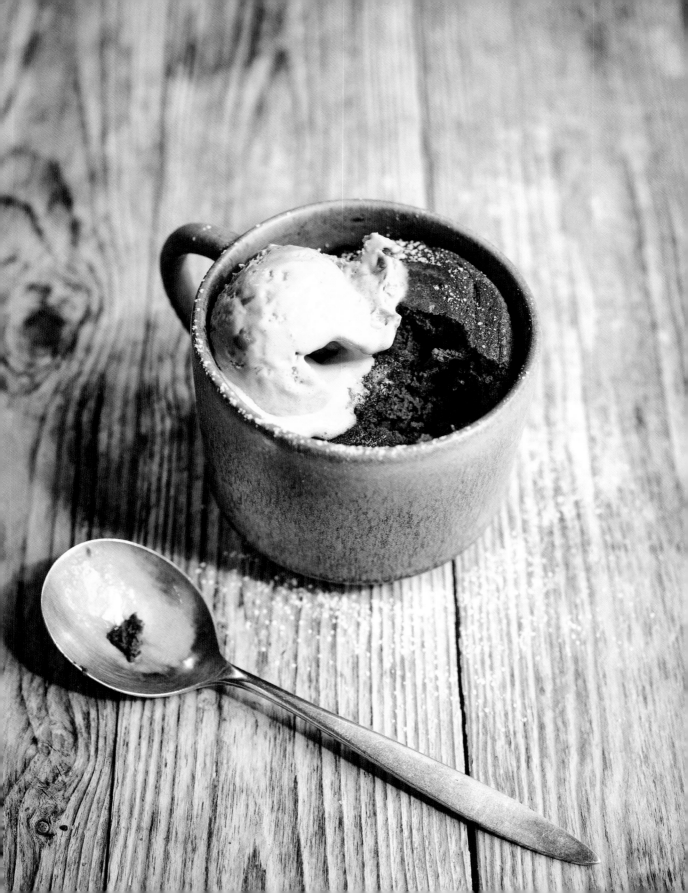

RASPBERRY MOUSSE WITH PEACHES

This has total peach melba vibes but with a fraction of the effort. You won't believe that whipping cream and raspberries in a blender would make the most delicate mousse in the world, but it's absolutely wonderful.

SERVES 2

300ml (10fl oz) double cream
150g (5oz) raspberries, reserving a couple to serve
handful of flaked almonds
1 ripe peach, cut into slices

1 In a blender, blitz the cream with most of the raspberries until thickened.

2 Divide among 2 bowls and top with the flaked almonds, the sliced peaches and the reserved raspberries.

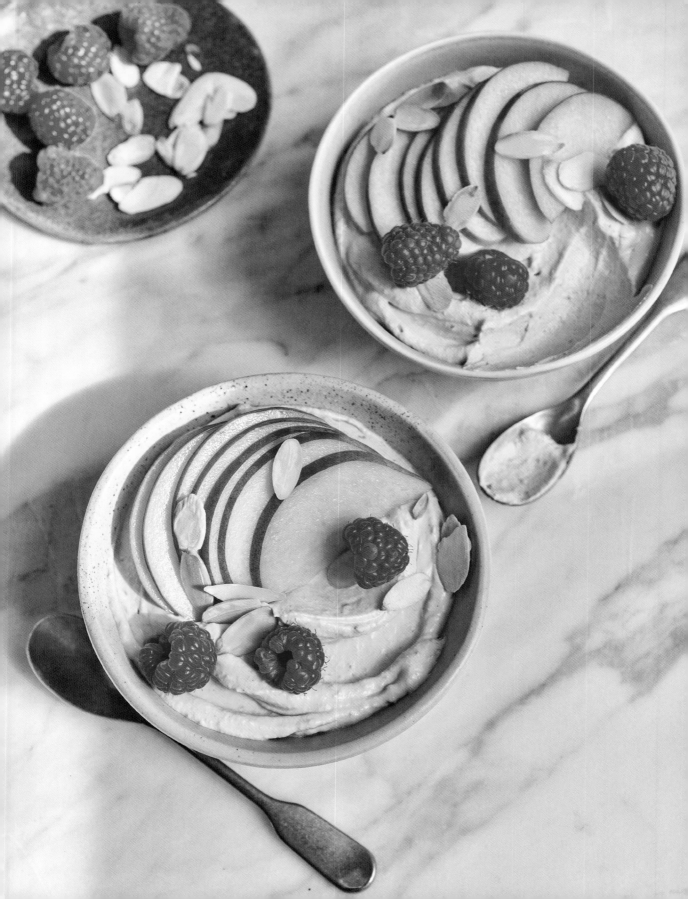

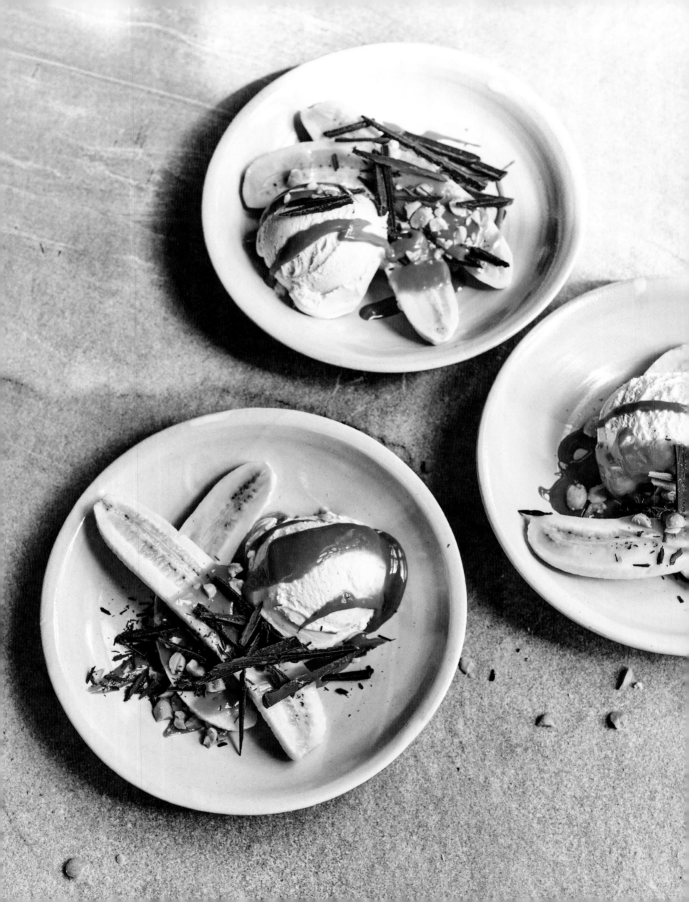

MISO BANANA SPLIT

I've only recently discovered miso paste, but, boy, does it pack a punch. Adding a few tablespoons of miso to shop-bought dulce de leche instantly makes this a super-fancy salted caramel sauce. Your mates will be so impressed, and it takes literally no effort at all. And the very best part: it involves zero cooking.

SERVES 4

2 tbsp miso paste
397g (14oz) tin of dulce de leche
4 bananas
4 scoops of vanilla ice cream
40g (1½oz) dark chocolate (70% cocoa solids), finely chopped
30g (1oz) salted peanuts, roughly chopped

1 Add the miso paste to the dulce de leche and stir well to combine – you can add more, if you like, to make it the perfect level of salted caramel to your taste.

2 Peel and halve the bananas and divide among four bowls.

3 Top each with a scoop of vanilla ice cream and the chopped chocolate and peanuts.

KIWI, LIME + GINGER NESTS

These little meringue tarts look unbelievably fancy for the amount of effort you're about to put in. This is a great little recipe to get the kids involved in. The stem ginger and kiwi is a really fantastic combination. I hope you enjoy them.

MAKES 8

300ml (10fl oz) double
  cream
zest of 2 limes
2 tbsp stem ginger syrup
8 meringue nests
3 kiwis, peeled and finely
  chopped
4 tsp stem ginger, finely
  chopped

1 Add the cream, zest of 1 lime and the stem ginger syrup to a large bowl and whisk with an electric whisk until soft peaks form.

2 Spoon a big dollop of cream into the centre of each meringue nest, top with some chopped kiwi and ½ teaspoon of chopped stem ginger.

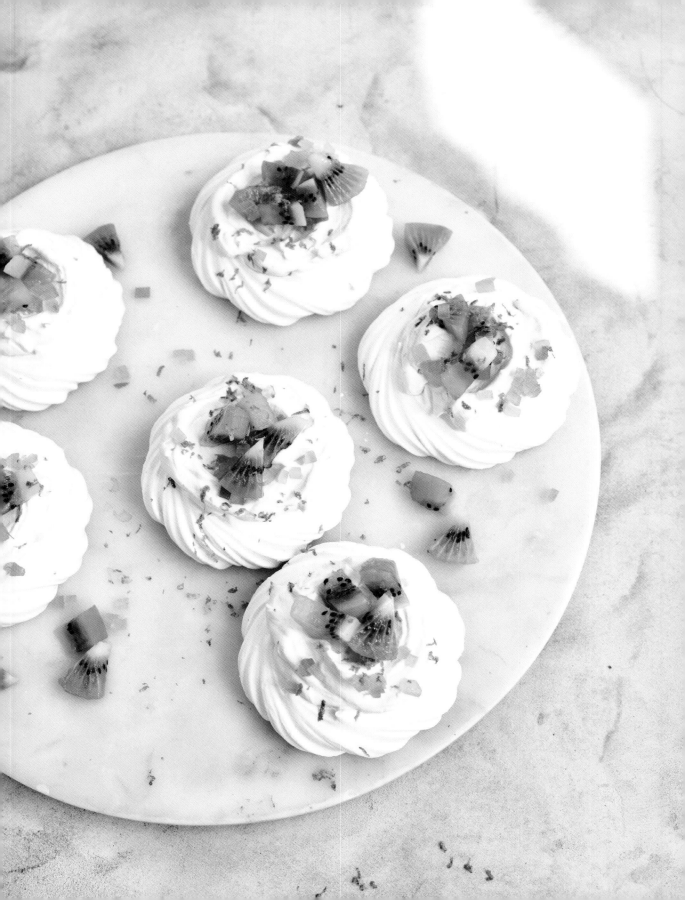

INSTANT CHOCOLATE MOUSSE

It's absolutely bonkers that you can make a chocolate mousse with no egg separating, no electric beaters and hardly any effort. Plus, there are only three ingredients. Madness! If you love a chocolate treat and have a sweet tooth like me, this recipe is for you.

SERVES 4

150g (5oz) marshmallows
350ml (12fl oz) whole milk
180g (6oz) dark chocolate
(70% cocoa solids),
chopped

1 Add the marshmallows and whole milk to a large saucepan (the mixture will expand!) and cook over a medium heat, stirring regularly until the marshmallows have melted and the mixture is lump-free. Make sure you're scraping along the bottom, ideally with a silicone spatula, so the mixture doesn't stick and burn.

2 Once the mixture has melted, tip in the chopped chocolate and turn off the heat. Give it one mix so that the marshmallow liquid is covering the chocolate, then leave to sit for 1–2 minutes to kick-start the chocolate melting. After 1 minute, mix thoroughly until smooth.

3 Pour the mixture into four moulds or glasses – it's ready to eat warm, or you can freeze it for 10 minutes, or refrigerate for at least an hour if you'd rather eat it cool or set.

TIP/SWAP
For even less effort, use chocolate chips to eliminate having to do any chopping!

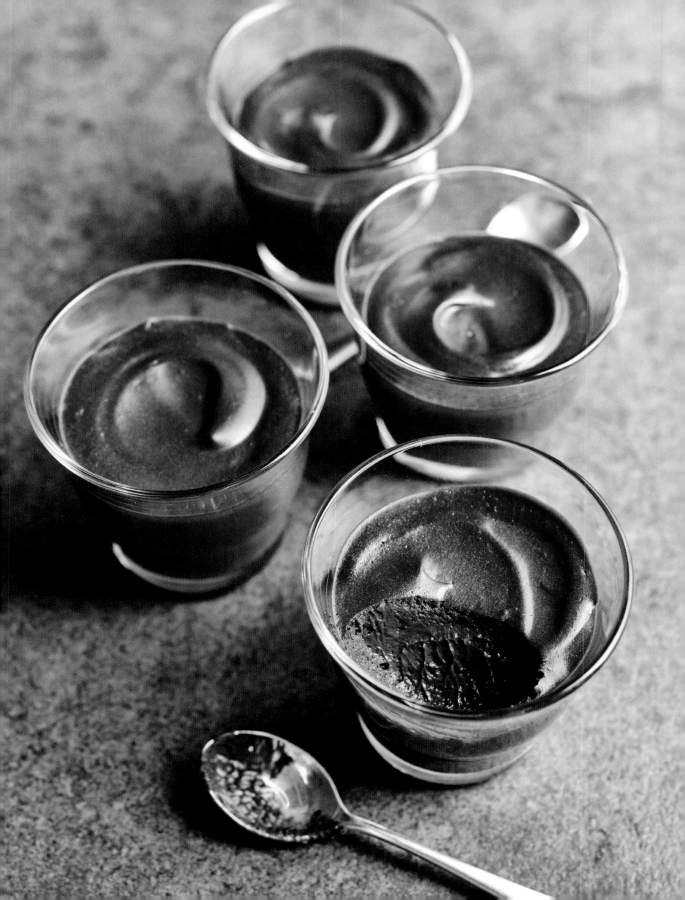

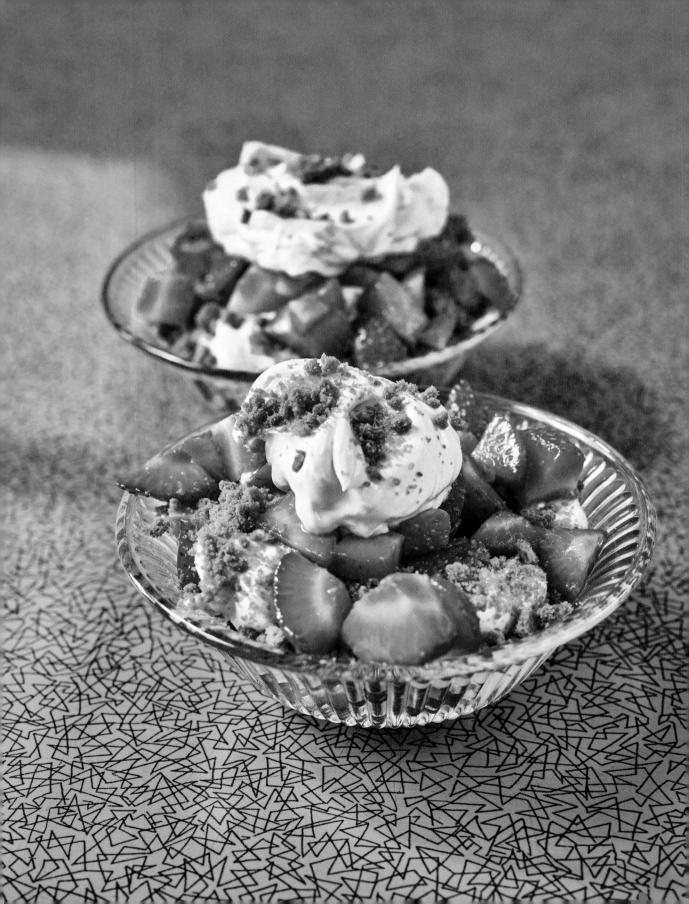

STRAWBERRY CHEESECAKE PARFAIT

V

This is a real showstopper to whip out at a dinner party or kids' birthday. No hanging around here for a cheesecake to set – I've taken all the good bits and made them into a lovely little layered dessert. Macerating the strawberries is an extra step but really worthwhile because it tastes delicious.

SERVES 2

100g (3½oz) strawberries, hulled and roughly chopped
1 tbsp caster sugar
100g (3½oz) cream cheese
100g (3½oz) natural yoghurt
3 ginger nut biscuits, bashed into crumbs

1 Add the strawberries and sugar to a bowl, mix, and leave to macerate for around 10–15 minutes.

2 Mix together the cream cheese and yoghurt in another bowl.

3 When ready to serve, create layers in a glass starting with the strawberries, then the cheese and yoghurt mix. Finally, sprinkle over the biscuit crumbs and serve.

STICKY RICE PUDDING WITH MANGO

You might think mango and sticky rice is a random combination, but it's proper dreamy. This super-speedy cheat's version makes the rice extra creamy and spoonable – much more like a rice pudding than you would traditionally find, but equally as delicious. Definitely try making this in mango season – you want the mango to be sweet, soft and fragrant, not hard and crunchy!

SERVES 2

250g (9oz) sachet of sticky rice or jasmine rice
400ml (14fl oz) tin of coconut milk
2 tbsp maple syrup
1 mango, peeled, stone removed and cut into slices
a few fresh mint sprigs, to serve
1 tbsp toasted sesame seeds
½ lime, cut into wedges

1 Add the rice and coconut milk to a medium saucepan and bring to a boil. Stir regularly while gently simmering for 8 minutes until the rice has plumped up and the milk is coating the rice grains and has significantly thickened (rather than soupy). Season to taste with maple syrup.

2 Serve topped with the mango slices, mint sprigs and sesame seeds, with a wedge of lime alongside to cut through the sweetness.

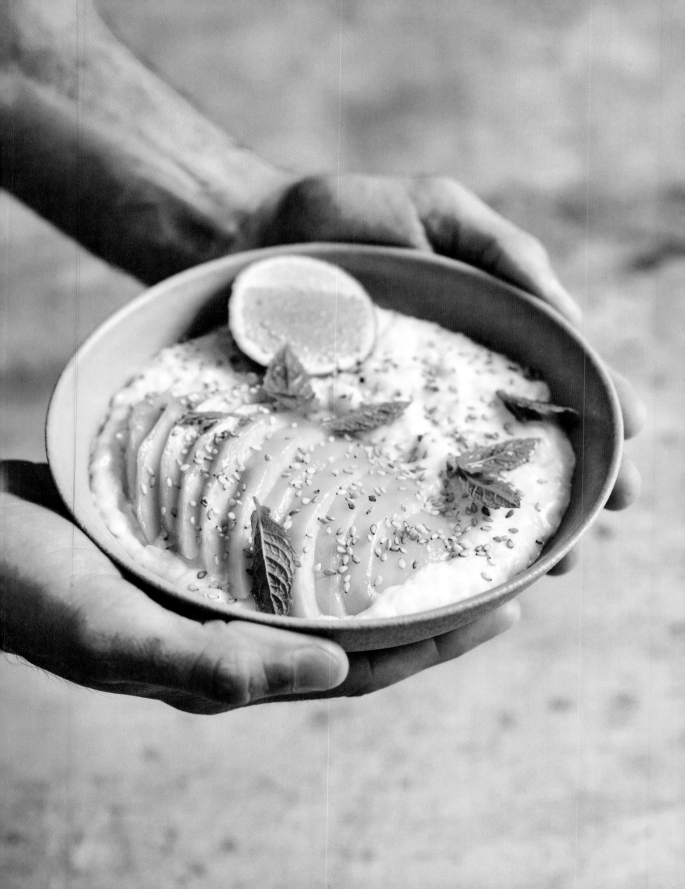

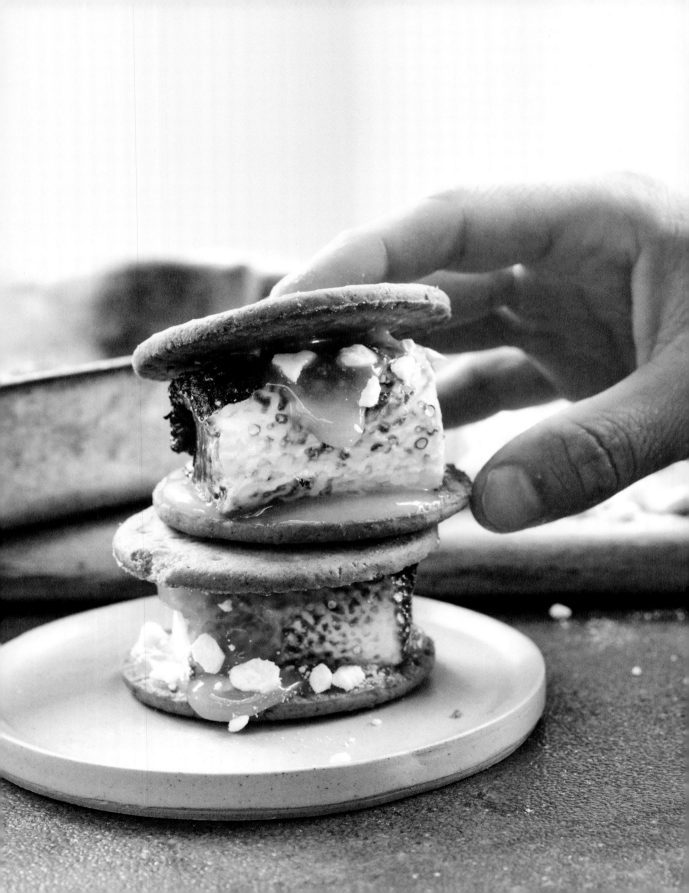

LEMON MERINGUE PIE SMORES

There's something so fun about toasting marshmallows. It takes me back to my childhood when we went camping and toasted them on an open fire. This is a lovely lemony twist on a smore, but it's a perfect treat to enjoy both indoors and outdoors.

SERVES 1

1 large marshmallow
2 digestive biscuits
1 tsp lemon curd
1 meringue kiss

1 Thread the marshmallow onto a metal skewer or fork, and turn on the gas hob. Rotate the skewer or fork regularly over the flame, using oven gloves, until scorched and melty.

2 Spread the lemon curd on one side of a biscuit, place the marshmallow on top in the middle, then crumble over the meringue kiss and sandwich with the other biscuit. Enjoy!

TIP/SWAP
This dish can be vegetarian if you use marshmallows without gelatine in them.

I always loved exercise, even from an early age. Looking back at my childhood now, I see that exercise was my release and my therapy. I found it hard to talk about my feelings and had things going on at home which I couldn't communicate to anyone about as a young boy. Through PE at school, I learned that I could release my anger, fear and anxiety by pushing myself physically. I connected the dots really early on and realised that I could calm myself down and change the way I felt in my head by doing something physical.

Exercise makes me feel happy and it's the main reason I still do it today without thought. It's just in my DNA and it's something I can't live without. Which is why I am so passionate about sharing this message and why I am especially driven to inspire young kids to fall in love with exercise and movement. It really does have powerful mental health benefits and will make you feel good. I hope this chapter helps you to take the first step towards fitness and therefore a happier mind too.

15-MINUTE WORKOUTS

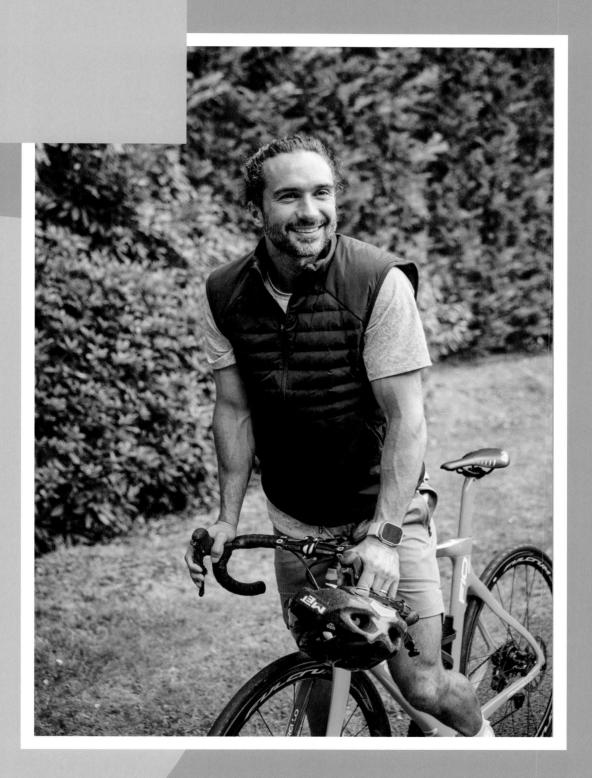

TRACKING YOUR PROGRESS

One thing that really helps me to feel good and stay motivated is setting goals and tracking my progress. For some people, they monitor their progress by seeing the weight loss on the scales, but I like to see my strength and fitness improve, so I keep a workout diary where I record my sessions. It becomes a record of all the hard work, sweat and effort you have put your body through. And that's something to be proud of.

CRUNCH THE NUMBERS

For cardio workouts, for example, I will keep track of the times I run, cycle or row over a certain distance. For strength sessions, I record the exercise name, the number of sets and reps, and the weights I use. This is one of the best tricks for breaking through a plateau and seeing strength gains. If you lift the same weights for the same number of reps and sets for months on end, you will not build muscle or strength. By recording the data, you can plan your sessions more effectively and focus on beating the numbers.

MOTIVATION

A workout diary is also a great motivational tool, especially for those times when your fat loss inevitably slows down or you feel like you are not seeing changes in the mirror. The numbers won't lie, and seeing how far you have come with your strength and fitness can really help you to stay focused and on track. It also just feels awesome to get stronger and you'll feel a sense of achievement and pride that far exceeds anything gained from doing a low-calorie diet.

WARMING UP AND COOLING DOWN

It is essential that you always warm up before any form of exercise, as well as cool down. These steps will ensure that you help to prevent any injuries and that you make your workout effective. You don't need to take long to do this, just a few minutes for each, but the stretching and movement in preparation and as an end, will really help you and your body.

BE PROUD OF ALL OF YOUR HARD WORK.

CREATE A PLAN

To make sure that I work all different parts of my body throughout the week and don't overfocus on one thing, I will spend 15 minutes at the beginning of my week creating a training plan. You might not stick to it completely, but it can be really helpful to have a visual aid. I have a whiteboard where I write my challenges for a particular workout or the details of my routine.

Below is an example of a weekly plan, but you can absolutely make this your own and repeat certain exercises over the days if this is your focus. Also, as you grow in confidence, strength, stamina and flexibility, and if you happen to find more time in the day, you might even be able to fit in multiple 15-minute routines on a single day.

A 15-MINUTE WEEKLY ROUTINE

DAY 1 Beginner HIIT Routine (see pages 166–170)

DAY 2 Abs Routine (see pages 190–194)

DAY 3 Lower Body Strength Routine
(see pages 183–187)

DAY 4 Upper Body Strength Routine
(see pages 178–182)

DAY 5 Advanced HIIT Routine (see pages 171–175)

DAY 6 Rest Day

DAY 7 Lower Body Mobility Routine
(see pages 198–203)

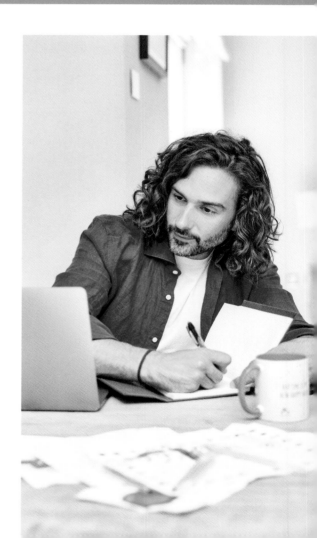

CHOOSING
THE RIGHT KIT

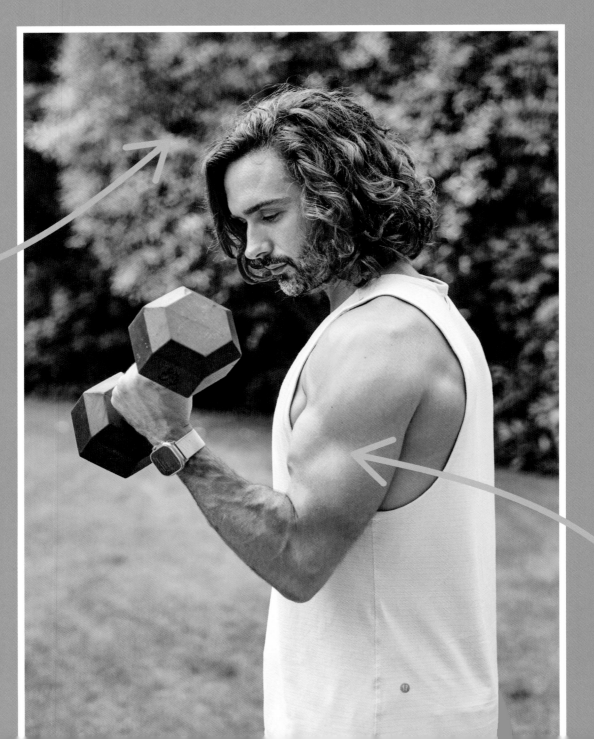

'WHAT HOME EQUIPMENT DO I NEED TO GET IN SHAPE?'

'HOW DO I KNOW WHAT WEIGHTS I SHOULD BUY?'

These are questions I get asked all the time, and here I'm going to share the key things that I always tell people.

STRENGTH

I always encourage people to start simple: start with body-weight exercises, especially if you're a beginner. It's important to build some foundational strength, fitness, coordination and balance first before you attempt to lift weights or invest in any expensive machines and equipment. Start with 1kg weights.

After that, I believe you can build a really strong physique with just your body and two pairs of dumbbells. I recommend a light pair (around 5kg) for upper body exercises, and a heavier set (around 10kg) for lower body moves. You can absolutely get by without an exercise bench – but if you can invest, do, as it will enable you to do a wider variety of moves.

CARDIO

In terms of home cardio equipment, my advice is this: if you hate running, don't buy a treadmill. If you love cycling, buy a bike. It's fundamentally important that you get some level of enjoyment out of whatever you buy, as otherwise it just becomes a very expensive clothes hanger or something you sell six months later. I bought a rower once thinking I would get into it and that it would help me get super-fit. But I hated rowing and I had never once chosen to do it at any gym I'd ever been to, so why would I have the motivation for it at home?

I BELIEVE YOU CAN BUILD A REALLY STRONG PHYSIQUE WITH JUST YOUR BODY AND TWO PAIRS OF DUMBBELLS.

MAKING TIME TO REST

Rest days are so important for the body. When we take time off to rest, we give our bodies a chance to repair and to grow. I factor in rest days every single week for recovery: I exercise hard every day for 5 days, followed by 1 full rest day where I do nothing – no cardio, no weights – and just relax.

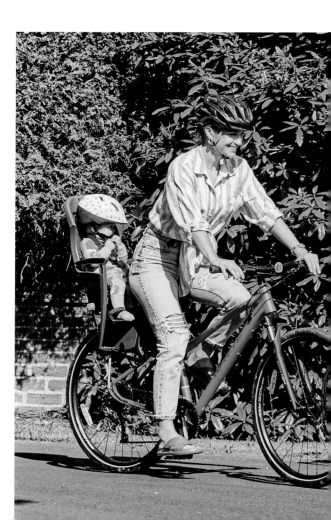

ACTIVE REST DAYS

On the seventh day, I might do something slightly easier like a mobility routine, or spend 15 minutes stretching and then maybe go for a walk or a gentle bike ride with the kids. I call this an active rest day because I'm moving but it's still a break from any high-intensity work.

LISTEN TO YOUR BODY

It's important to listen to your body, too. If after a full week of training you are feeling run down, exhausted or achy, drop back a bit and take a day or two off, or consider reducing the number of times you train per week. You may find that for your body and lifestyle, three workouts spaced out throughout the week is perfect for you. The main thing is to check in with yourself, make adjustments if necessary and focus on doing what feels good.

BEING INJURED

Being injured is the worst. For the past few years, it has felt like I'm always injured somewhere. It's as if my injuries just move from one body part to the next. It can be very frustrating, particularly if you have an ongoing issue that you can't shake off.

If you're struggling with an injury, my advice is to try not to train through it and instead to rest it. Properly resting can be one of the hardest things to do, especially if, like me, you love to train and it's a big part of your daily life and what makes you happy. But rest is essential, so take some time off, let any swelling or inflammation go down and, if you can, book an appointment with a doctor or a physio as soon as possible. It won't be cheap, but one hour with a good physio can really speed up the recovery process and allow you to get back to training sooner.

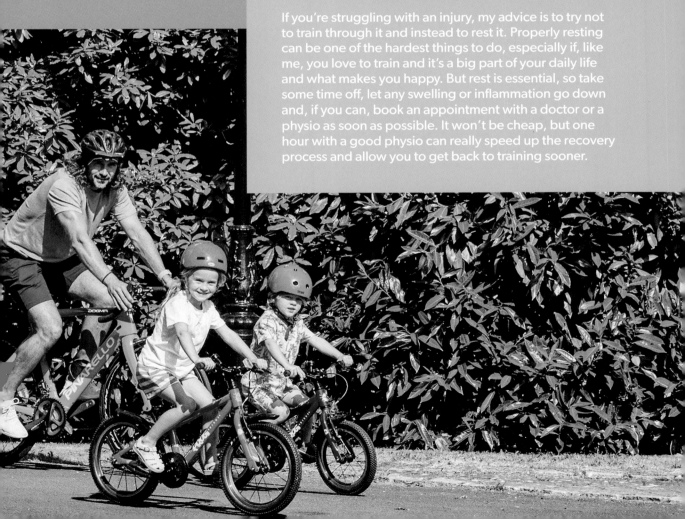

MOVEMENT

Nothing has the ability to shift your mental state as quickly and as effectively as physical exercise. This doesn't mean you have to find an hour a day to do a full gym session or complete a super-intense workout: all movement is positive, and 15 minutes is a great place to start.

Fifteen minutes really can be just enough time to boost your energy, clear your mind and leave you feeling more motivated. Once you commit to doing something physical, the release of endorphins feels so wonderful you will want to do more. It suddenly becomes 25 or 30 minutes and you feel energised and fantastic. It all comes down to reminding yourself how much better you will feel afterwards and taking that first step to get moving.

Movement is anything that gets you moving your body, working your muscles and using some energy. It's so important to try different types of movement until you find one that feels good and that sticks. This could be anything from walking, hiking, swimming, cycling, completing a HIIT session, lifting weights, yoga, indoor climbing, aerobics class, roller skating, gardening, playing hide-and-seek or even climbing trees in the park – you name it.

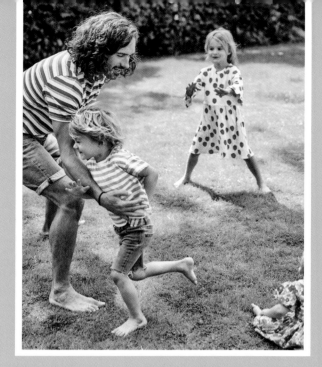

I am a huge fan of home workouts, especially for people with kids or busy work lives. Anything that reduces the friction and the barriers to participation is a good thing, because it means you are more likely to fit it in and stick with it. It would be amazing if we all had the money and hours in the day to attend a fully equipped gym with a trainer, but for the majority that's just not realistic. Even those who can financially afford gym memberships often struggle to go consistently because life gets in the way.

If you can turn your living room or garden into your workout space, the excuses start to fade away. Even with young kids or a hectic workday, you can almost always find 15 minutes. To help you get started, I have designed two simple 15-minute bodyweight home workouts for you. They require no equipment and very little space to complete. Have fun!

15-MINUTE BEGINNER HIIT ROUTINE

This is a classic bodyweight workout designed with some basic moves for beginners. 'HIIT' stands for High Intensity Interval Training and involves short bursts of effort followed by a rest. Aim to do each exercise for 30 seconds, followed by a 30-second rest between each move. Repeat the circuit 3 times. One thing you can be certain of is that you always feel better afterwards.

1

JOG ON THE SPOT

A. March, jog or sprint as fast as you can and on the spot for 30 seconds. Keep your back straight and drive your knees up as high as you can.

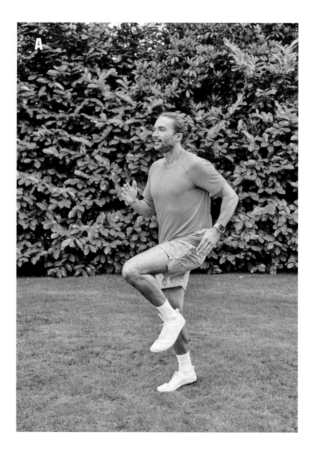

2 SQUATS

A. Stand with your feet about shoulder-width apart.

B. Slowly bend at the knees, as if you are sitting down on a chair. Sit down as low as you can comfortably go while keeping your feet flat on the ground. Then, drive your weight into your heels and begin to straighten your legs into a full standing position.

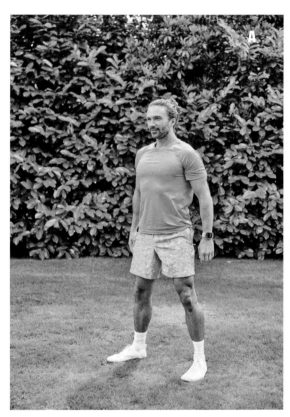
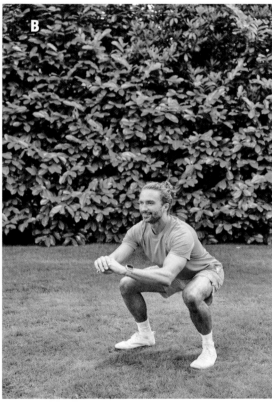

YOU WILL NEVER REGRET A WORKOUT; YOU CAN ALWAYS FIND 15 MINUTES TO EXERCISE AND HAVE FUN.

3 KNEE SMASHERS

A. Stand up straight. Begin by lifting your arms straight and directly up above your head.

B. Drive your knees up above your hips one at a time and bring the hands down towards each knee as you do so. Try to do this as fast as you can. You will feel your heart rate elevate rapidly.

THIS IS A GREAT ONE TO RAISE THE HEART RATE.

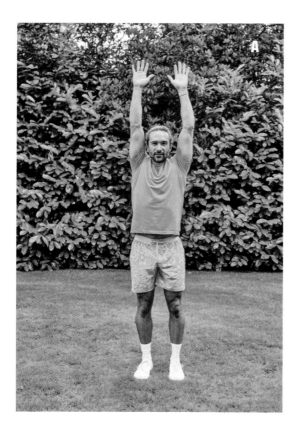

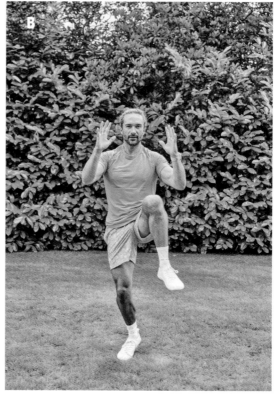

AN AWESOME MOVE FOR BUILDING STRONG GLUTES AND THIGHS.

4 REVERSE LUNGES

A. Start with your feet together and back straight.

B. Step your right leg straight back behind you and bend the knee, lowering it towards the ground. Maintain good balance and slowly drive through your left heel to bring yourself back to the starting position. Repeat this for 30 seconds, alternating between legs.

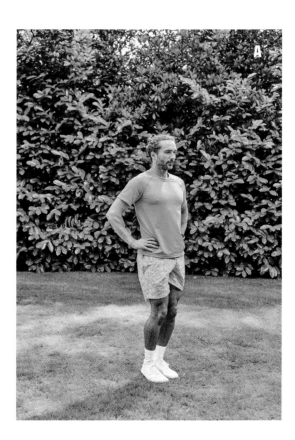

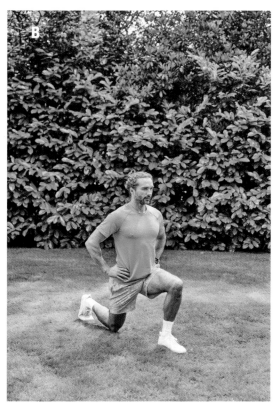

GET READY TO GET A GOOD SWEAT ON.

5 MOUNTAIN CLIMBERS

A. Start in a high plank position with your hands stacked under your shoulders.

B. Drive your knees up towards your chest one at a time. Do this as fast as you can. Keep your arms and back as straight as possible.

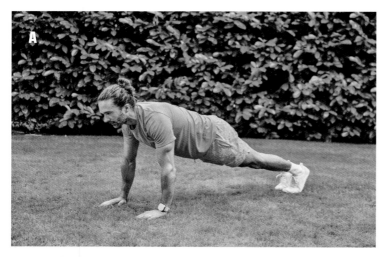

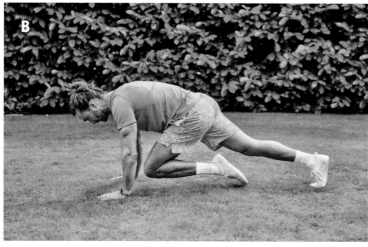

15-MINUTE ADVANCED HIIT ROUTINE

This is a more advanced bodyweight session and a great high-intensity workout when you are short on time but still want to get a good sweat on. This will get your muscles burning, that's for sure. Aim to work for 40 seconds on each exercise, with a 20-second rest between moves. Repeat the circuit 3 times for a total of 15 minutes of intense effort. Good luck.

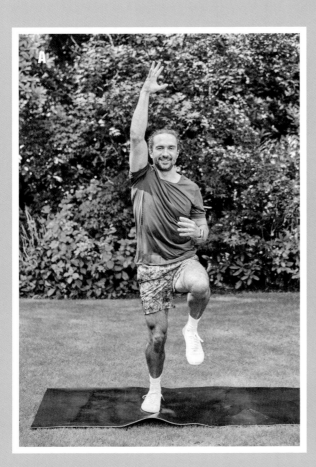

1

CLIMB THE ROPE

A. Sprint on the spot. As you do this, lift your arms above your head and pull an imaginary rope down towards your waist. Pump the arms and knees up as high as you can and as fast as possible.

2

PUSH-UPS

A. Do these from a full press-up position or with your knees resting on the floor for an easier version. Focus on bending at the elbows and lowering your chest to the floor.

B. Push yourself back up until your arms are straight. Do this move slowly and with control to increase the intensity.

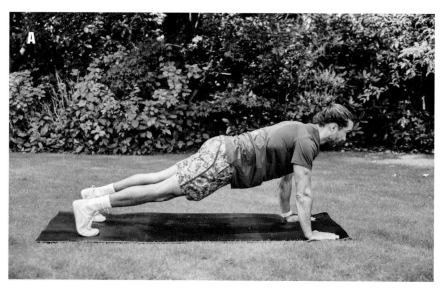

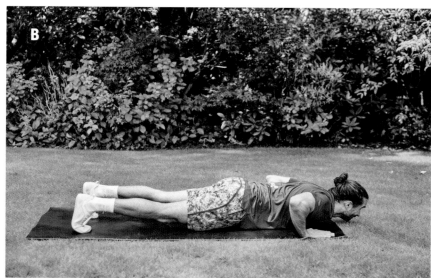

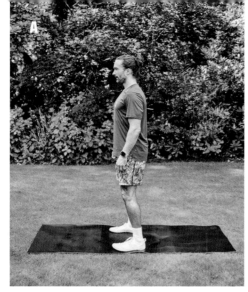

3

SQUAT JUMPS

A. Start in a standing position with your feet flat on the ground.

B. Bending at the knees, lower yourself into a low squat position.

C. Then explode upwards, using your legs to lift your feet off the ground. Land as gently as possible, like a spring. Repeat these squat jumps for 40 seconds. Leg burner!

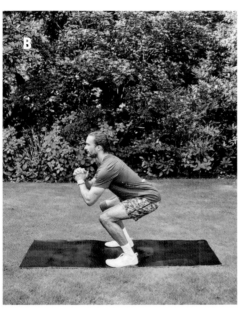

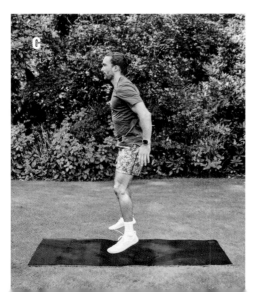

THESE SQUAT JUMPS WILL GET YOUR MUSCLES BURNING.

4

SIDE THRUSTERS

A. Start in a high plank position with your hands stacked under your shoulders.

B. Jump both feet up and out towards your elbows. Jump the feet back to the start position and repeat, quickly alternating from the left to the right.

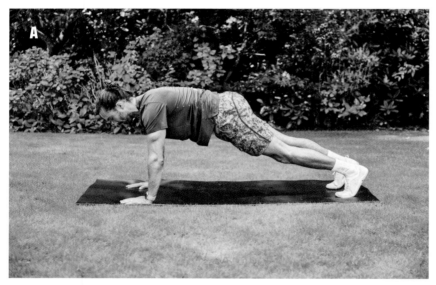

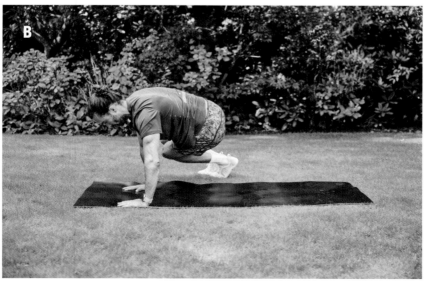

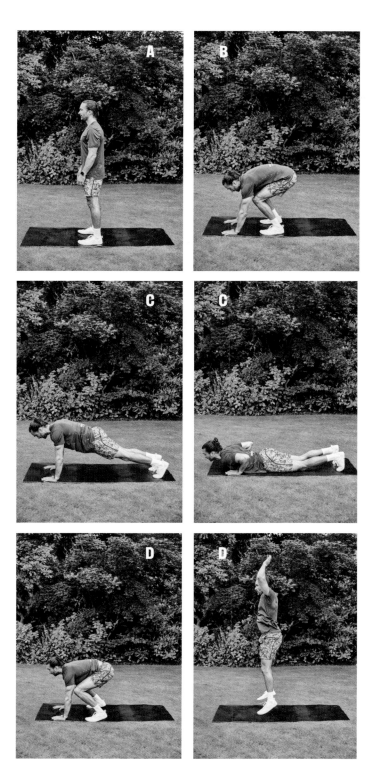

5

BURPEES

A. Start in a standing position.

B. Bend forwards and place both hands on the ground.

C. Kick your legs back into a high plank, then lower your chest to the ground.

D. Push up, jump your legs back up towards your hands and stand up straight, jumping slightly off the ground. Repeat this up-and-down movement for 40 seconds.

LOVE THEM OR HATE THEM, BURPEES ARE VERY GOOD AT RAISING YOUR HEART RATE AND BURNING ENERGY.

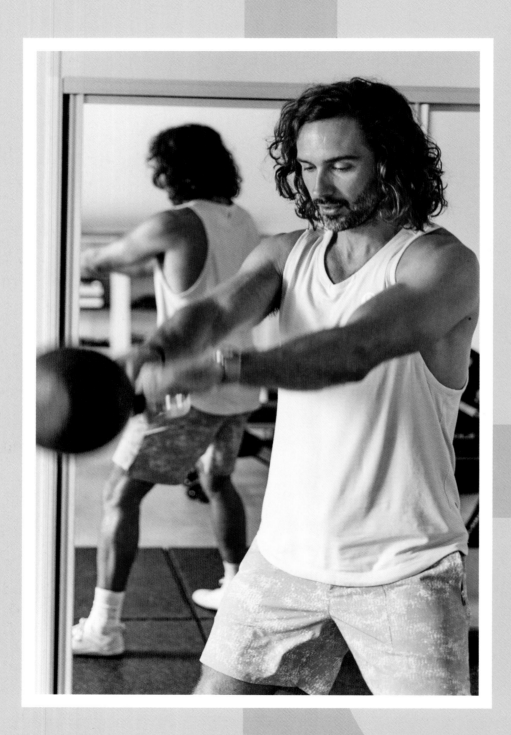

STRENGTH

There really is nothing greater than feeling strong. If your goal is to get toned or lean, this means you want to be strong and increase your muscle mass. In order to build and maintain lean muscle, we need to focus on resistance training. Lifting weights increases strength, improves bone density and heart health, helps manage blood sugar levels and helps your body metabolise body fat. This is because muscle burns more energy than body fat, so the more lean muscle you have, the more calories your body will be burning at rest. Not only will strength training have you feeling good physically, it can also really help with your mental strength and resilience. It really can lift the weight of stress off your shoulders and help you release any anger or frustration from your mind.

I have designed two resistance training sessions for you to try at home. All you need to complete the workouts is a pair of dumbbells. One workout is focused on the upper body and one is focused on the lower body. The most important thing when lifting weights is to focus on your form and technique. Lift with good control and a slow tempo to stabilise your joints and reduce the risk of injury. It's a good idea to start with a lower weight to get the correct form and gradually increase it as you get stronger.

15-MINUTE UPPER BODY STRENGTH ROUTINE

1 BICEP CURLS

A. Stand with one dumbbell in each hand.

B. Keeping elbows tight against the body, curl and rotate the dumbbell up towards your shoulder. Alternate on each side, slowly controlling the weight on the way up and down.

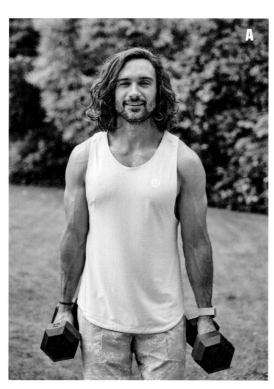
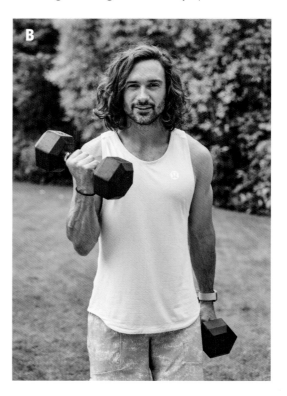

Building muscle increases strength, reduces the risk of injury, improves our metabolism and builds our confidence. It's hard work but it's worth it, and if fat loss is your goal, then resistance training is essential. All you need for this 15-minute workout is a pair of dumbbells and a chair. Start with light weights and gradually increase them as you get stronger. The last 2–3 repetitions of each exercise should feel challenging, but you should still be able to complete them with good form.

CONTINUE EACH EXERCISE FOR 60 SECONDS AND THEN MOVE STRAIGHT ONTO THE NEXT MOVE WITH NO REST. REPEAT THE CIRCUIT 3 TIMES.

2 SHOULDER PRESS

A. Stand with a dumbbell in each hand. Press the weights up directly above your head.

B. Lower the weights slowly until there is a 90-degree bend at the elbow and tension on the deltoid muscles. Repeat with good control for a full minute.

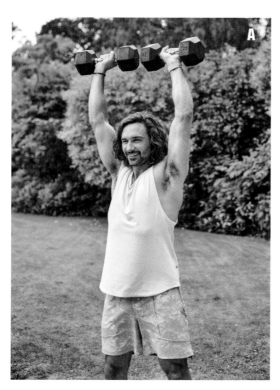 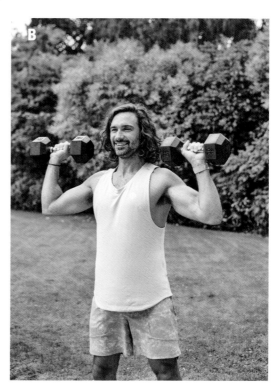

3

BENT-OVER ROWS

A. Stand with one dumbbell in each hand. Bend the knees gently and lean forwards slightly towards the floor.

B. Using the muscles in your back and arms, squeeze and pull the dumbbells up towards your torso. Visualise squeezing your shoulder blades together. Slowly lower them back down until your arms are straight, and repeat.

THESE ARE HARD WORK BUT THEY'RE SO WORTH IT.

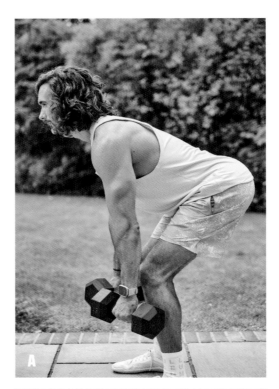

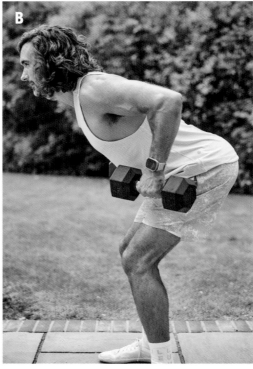

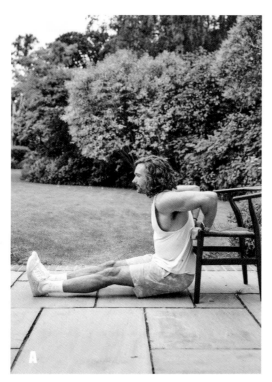

4

TRICEP DIPS ON A CHAIR

A. Place your hands on a chair, bench or a step behind you. Slowly bend at the elbows, lowering your bottom towards the floor.

B. When your elbows are bent to 90 degrees, push yourself back up until your arms are straight. Keep your back close to the chair and your elbows tucked in against the body.

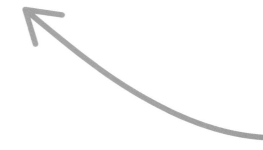

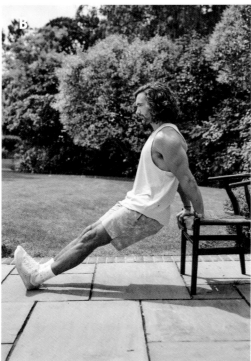

THIS EXERCISE CAN ALSO BE DONE ON A BENCH IF YOU HAVE ONE.

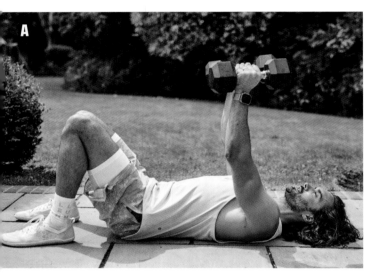

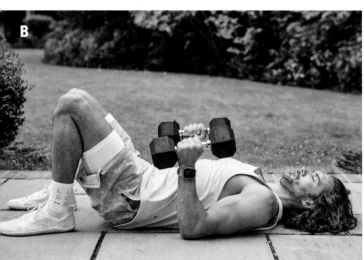

5

DUMBBELL FLOOR PRESS

A. Lie flat on the floor with your knees bent and feet on the floor. Hold one dumbbell in each hand and press them up directly above you.

B. Keeping the elbows close to the body, bend the elbows and lower the weights towards your body. Press up again and repeat the move slowly for a minute.

15-MINUTE LOWER BODY STRENGTH ROUTINE

Time to build the lower body. This circuit focuses on the quadriceps, glutes and hamstrings. Aim to complete each exercise for 40 seconds with a 20-second rest between moves. Repeat the circuit 3 times. Do each move as slowly and with as much control as possible with a weight that challenges you.

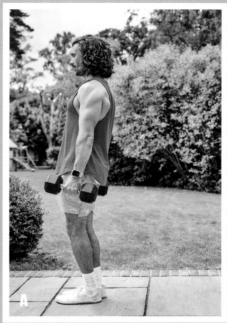

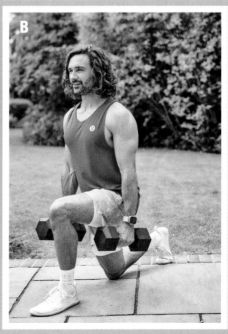

1 REVERSE LUNGES

A. Hold a dumbbell in each hand. Start with your feet together and back straight.

B. Step your right leg straight back behind you and bend the knee, lowering it towards the ground. Maintaining good balance, slowly drive through your left heel to bring yourself back to the starting position. Repeat this for 30 seconds, alternating between legs.

THIS EXERCISE FOCUSES ON THE HAMSTRINGS AND GLUTES.

2 ROMANIAN DEAD LIFTS (RDLS)

A. Hold one dumbbell in each hand, stand straight.

B. Lean over slightly with softly bent knees. Keep your back straight and lower the dumbbells towards the ground. When you feel a stretch in the hamstrings (usually just below the knees), pull the dumbbells back up until your legs are straight. Repeat slowly.

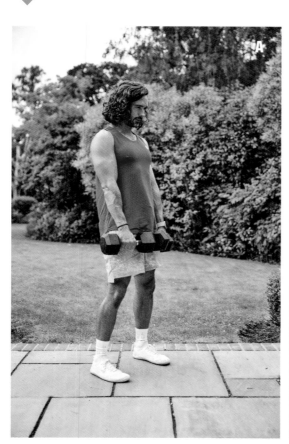

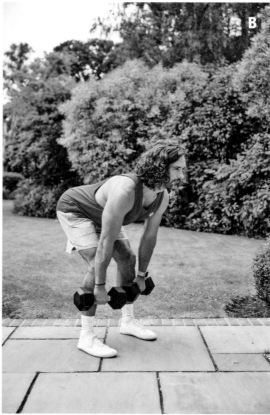

3 FRONT SQUATS

A. Hold one dumbbell in each hand and rack them up by your shoulders. Stand with your feet about a shoulder-width apart.

B. Lower yourself down by bending at the knees. Focus on keeping your back straight, core engaged, elbows up and feet flat on the ground. Drive through the heels into a standing position and repeat.

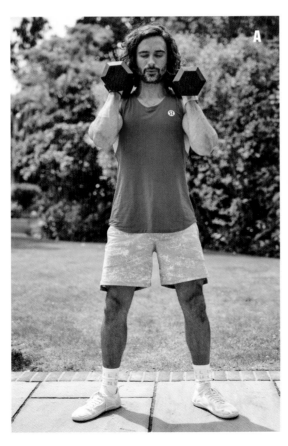

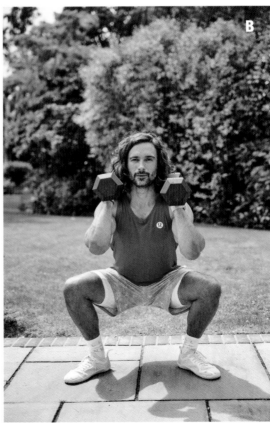

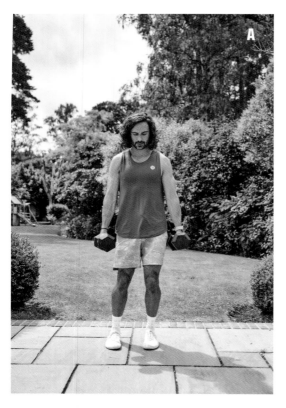

4

LATERAL LUNGES

A. Hold one dumbbell in each hand. Stand with feet together and hang the weights down by your side.

B. Step out to the side in a lateral movement, bending at the knee. You will feel a big stretch on the inside of the straight leg, so take it slow and steady and go only as far as you feel comfortable. Repeat on the other leg for 40 seconds before taking a rest.

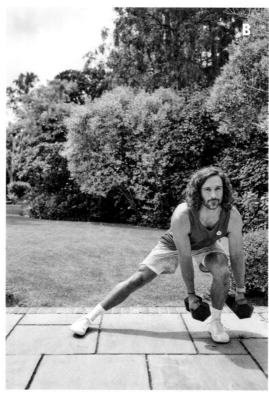

5 WEIGHTED GLUTE BRIDGE

A. Lie on the floor with your head and shoulders on the ground, your knees bent and your feet flat on the ground. Place a dumbbell on your waist and drive both feet firmly into the ground.

B. Using your glutes, drive your hips up off the ground. Slowly lower yourself down and repeat, focusing on squeezing your glutes as much as possible.

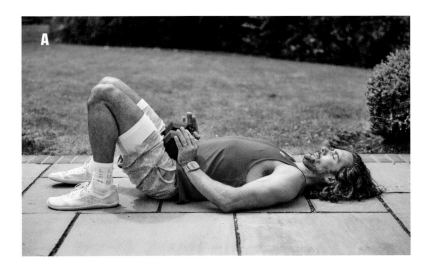

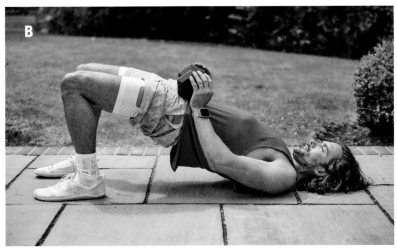

THIS IS ONE OF MY FAVOURITE GLUTE EXERCISES.

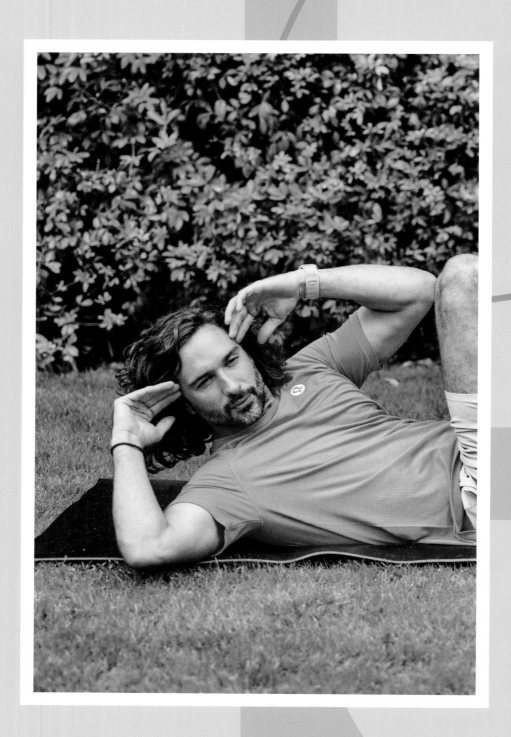

ABS

Everyone loves a little abs workout. It's always nice to feel strong in the core and it can really improve your posture and help you get the most out of other exercises too. The routine I have created for you here can be done by itself, but remember if you want to be able to visibly see your abs you need to reduce your body fat, and that will only come from a consistent diet and doing the more intense full-body workouts, so aim to get those done during the week too.

My suggestion, if you have the time, is to add the abs circuit onto the end of one of your full body workouts 2–3 times a week. But this can also be done on its own when lying on the floor watching your favourite TV show. Just focus on good breathing and fully contracting your abdominal muscles. I find closing my eyes and really focusing on the mind and muscle connection can help. Avoid holding your hands behind your neck and pulling from there because this will only hurt your neck and you won't feel it in the abs.

15-MINUTE ABS ROUTINE

This is my favourite abs circuit and I usually bolt it on to the end of a HIIT or strength workout (see pages 166–175 and/or 178–187). Complete each exercise for 40 seconds, rest for 20 seconds, then move onto the next one. Aim to repeat the circuit 3 times for a total of 15 minutes. Good luck.

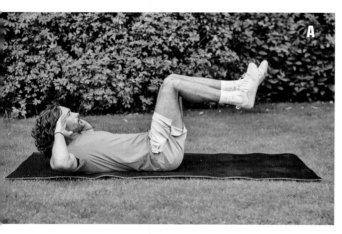

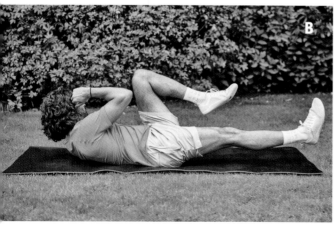

1

BICYCLE CRUNCHES

A. Start by lying flat on your back. Lift both of your legs up off the ground and bend at 90 degrees. Resting your hands behind your head or at your temples, crunch your head and shoulders up off the ground.

B. Twist your right elbow towards your left knee using your abs. Slowly kick the right foot away from you until your leg is fully extended. Alternate each side. Do this exercise as slowly as possible to really activate the abs.

EVERYONE LOVES A LITTLE ABS WORKOUT.

2 SINGLE LEG CRUNCH

A. Start by lying flat on your back with your feet on the floor and knees bent. Raise your arms straight up above your head.

B. Slowly crunch up and as you do, raise one leg straight up towards your body. The aim is to touch the foot or shin with both hands. Repeat, slowly alternating each leg as you crunch up off the floor.

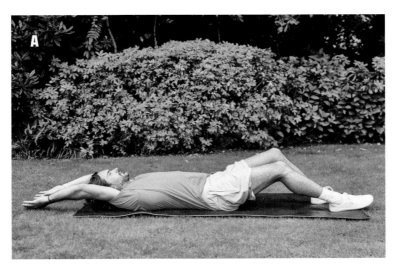

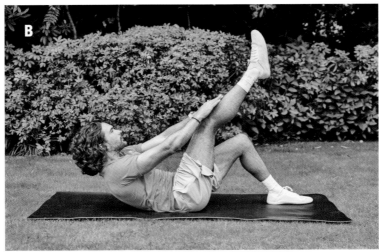

THIS IS A TOUGH EXERCISE BUT IT'S VERY GOOD FOR STRENGTHENING YOUR OBLIQUE MUSCLES.

3

SIDE PLANK

A. Place your right elbow on the floor directly underneath your right shoulder. Keeping your feet together and legs as straight as possible, lift your hips up off the ground. Reach your right arm straight up above your head and hold this static position for 20 seconds. Rotate around and complete the same on the left elbow for 20 seconds.

B. Alternatively, you can complete the same movement with your legs bent at the knees.

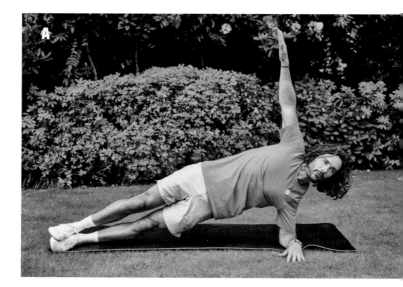

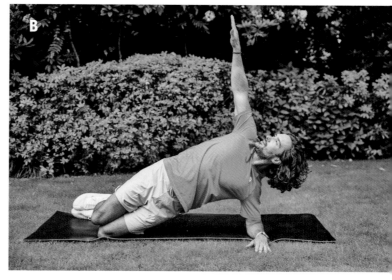

SLOW-MO MOUNTAIN CLIMBERS

A. Start in a high plank position with hands stacked under the shoulders. Keep a strong core with your spine straight and hold that position.

B. From there, slowly drive one knee up as high as possible towards your chin to feel your abs activate. Pause for a second, then slowly return the leg to its starting position. Alternate between each leg and keep the movement as slowly as possible.

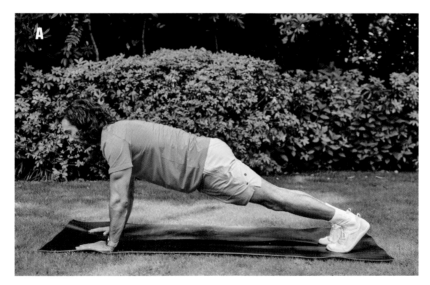

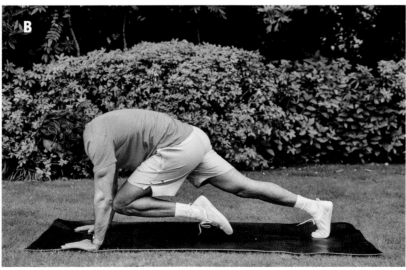

5 ELBOW PLANK/SPIDER VARIATION

A. Start in a basic plank position with elbows stacked under the shoulders and your back flat. Engage your core and draw your belly button up towards your spine. Hold this static for 40 seconds while inhaling and exhaling slowly.

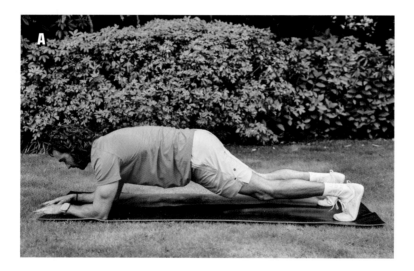

B. To increase the intensity, bring one knee at a time up towards your elbow. This will send you off balance and engage the obliques.

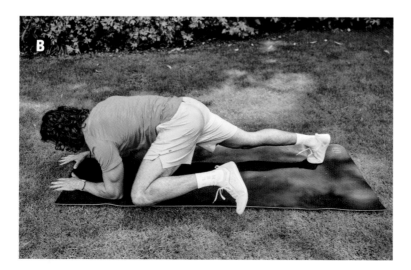

USE THESE 15-MINUTE, FEEL-GOOD ROUTINES WHENEVER AND WHEREVER YOU CAN. FIND WHAT WORKS FOR YOU AND STICK WITH IT.

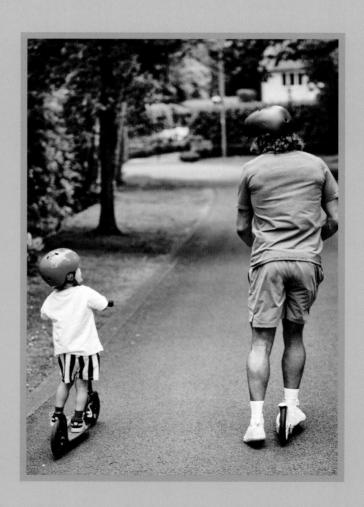

MOBILITY

If only I had listened to this next piece of advice sooner. It has taken me a long time to come to terms with the importance of regular mobility work and how necessary it is if you want to have a happy body that is pain- and injury-free. I used to be able to get away with training super-hard and consistently without much stretching or recovery work, but with each year that passes I have had to adapt and prioritise this work.

I find the exercise part of a workout more enjoyable than stretching, flexibility and mobility. I find it boring and it can also be very uncomfortable. But in order for me to stay pain-free I have to do a few specific stretches every day and I'm finally in the habit of doing it daily. Taking your hips or shoulders through full controlled rotations each day keeps the range of motion and your joints healthy.

In all honesty, the only reason I started to commit to this stuff was because I was in regular pain and discomfort during my workouts. It's only after years of not feeling good in my body and having a slight pain in my hip when I did any form of squat or lunge that I decided I needed to do something. It's quite common for people to wait until they are injured or in pain to start thinking about mobility, but don't do what I did. Think about your body holistically and think about your future self. Rather than waiting for your body to break down and only then remedying it, think about prevention.

I have tried everything from physio and osteopathy to acupuncture and deep-tissue massage, which do help in the short term, but nothing has had a greater impact on my pain than consistent mobility work. It really has changed my life. It's the next tip I'm about to share that has had the most impact for me.

The only way I've been able to get this daily work done with any consistency is by bolting it onto something else. I find it much easier to stretch when I'm distracted, so I usually do most of my stretching when I'm on an online call or watching TV. It may seem like a crazy idea to be stretching while on a call, but no one cares and it's so beneficial to your body. Imagine if every time you had a 30-minute online meeting you used that time to stretch your hip flexors. Or when you watched your favourite TV show, you sat on the floor and stretched your glutes in the pigeon pose rather than sitting all folded up on the sofa. Trust me, it works, and it's so much easier to fit in when you combine it with another task, because you can do it more often and without much effort.

I have created two active mobility routines. One focuses on the lower body, including the hips, and the other focuses on the joints of the upper body. If you are like me and suffer with tight hips and glutes and lower back pain, these will change your life.

15-MINUTE LOWER BODY MOBILITY ROUTINE

If you want smooth and buttery hips, then this routine is right up your street. These six moves have quite literally transformed my body. I do this routine regularly and I'm now pain-free, I'm able to move better and I'm getting more out of my workouts because of my new and improved range of motion.

This isn't a static series of moves where you sit and hold a stretch. This is more active: each exercise incorporates gentle movement to open the joints and increase strength in that range of movement. Aim to spend around 2 minutes on each move (1 minute per side). Move at a slow, controlled pace and focus on big inhales and exhales as you relax the muscles and take the stretch deeper. You can do this routine at the start or end of a workout, or both if you really want to feel the benefits. It's not easy to begin with and some moves may feel uncomfortable, but stick with it and you will feel amazing.

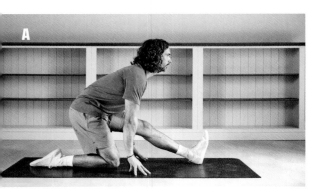

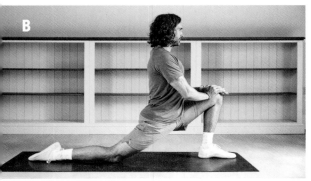

1 HIP FLEXOR/HAMSTRING STRETCH

A. Start by kneeling down on your right knee and stretching your left leg out in front of you.

B. Place your hands on your left knee and slowly lean forwards into a low lunge position. This will create a nice, deep stretch in your right hip flexor. Stay here for a couple of seconds, then gently rock backwards, sitting back into your right heel, keeping your left leg as straight as possible. This will create a deep stretch in your left hamstring. Repeat this back-and-forward movement for 1 minute, and then repeat on the other side.

2 SPIDER CLIMBER/T-OPEN

A. Start in a high plank position.

B. Step your right foot up beside your right hand.

C. Take your right hand off the ground and rotate your arm up towards the sky to form a letter T. Slowly rotate back down and return the hand to the ground. Step your right foot back into the high plank position and repeat for the left side. Repeat this for 2 minutes.

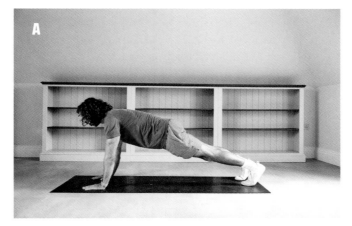

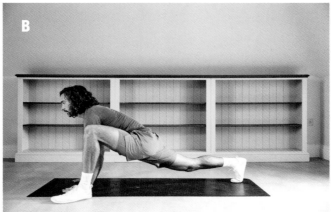

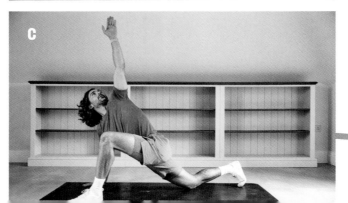

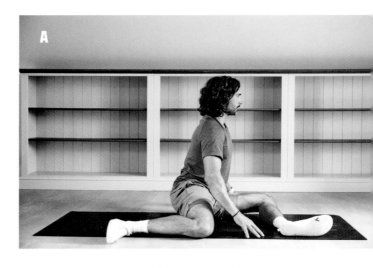

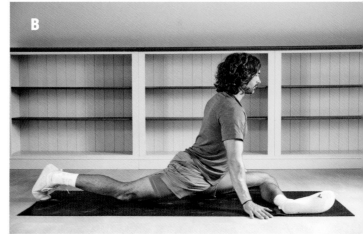

THIS IS MY FAVOURITE MOVE IN THE WORLD. IT'S THE ULTIMATE FOR YOUR HIPS.

3

90/90 SIT/PIGEON POSE

A. Beginners should start with the 90/90 sit. Sit on the floor and try to form a 90-degree angle with the front and back legs. Alternatively, you might like to try the pigeon pose, extending the back leg out behind you.

B. Lean slightly forwards and bring your chest towards the ground. Focus on driving the front knee and foot into the ground, creating an external rotation of the hip. Sit here in this stretch for 30 seconds, then switch legs and complete on the other side. Repeat two rounds on each leg.

NB. For the pigeon pose, you can spend the first 30 seconds just relaxing into the stretch, and then actively drive the knee and foot into the ground for the final 30 seconds.

SEATED HIP ROTATIONS

A. Sit on the ground with your legs bent and feet placed wide apart. Place your arms on the floor behind you to support yourself.

B. Using the muscles in your hips, actively drive one knee down towards the floor as much as possible without your bottom coming off the ground. Then drive the same knee back towards the wall behind you with as much range as possible. Repeat slowly on each side for 2 minutes in total.

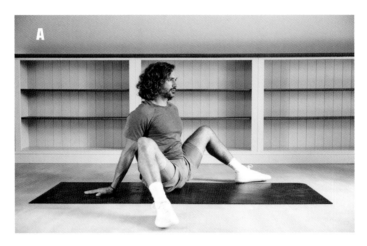

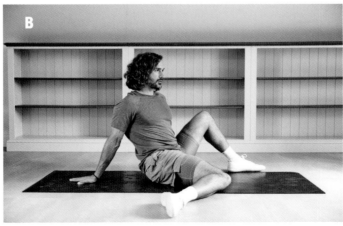

ANOTHER GREAT HIP OPENER.

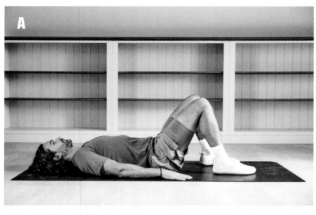

5

THREAD THE NEEDLE

A. Start by lying flat on the ground with your knees bent and both feet on the floor.

B. Place your right foot across your left knee.

C. Thread your hand through the gap and hug the left knee towards you. Hold it for 1 minute and repeat on the other side.

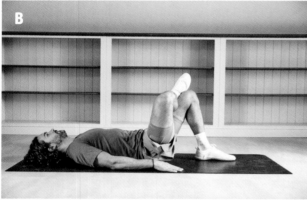

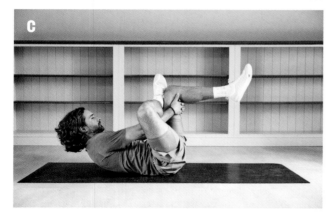

THIS IS ANOTHER STRONG HIP OPENER I LEARNED IN YOGA.

THIS IS A GREAT MOVE TO FINISH ON AND BRING IT ALL TOGETHER.

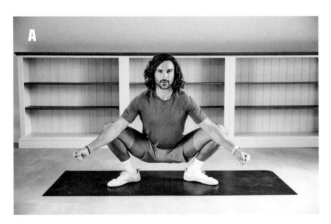

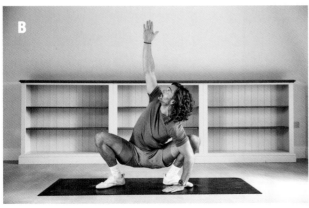

6

DEEP SQUAT/T-OPEN

A. Place your feet in a comfortable position that allows you to sit into a low, deep squat while keeping your heels flat on the ground. Try to keep a neutral spine and slowly lower yourself towards the ground. If this is enough of a stretch, stay here for 2 minutes.

B. For an extra challenge and a deeper stretch, try to keep one hand on the ground and bring the other arm right up above the head. If you can manage this, slowly alternate each arm while focusing on your breathing.

15-MINUTE UPPER BODY MOBILITY ROUTINE

This is a great routine to improve your upper body mobility, especially around the shoulder joint and scapula. If you experience any tightness in your neck or shoulders, or you struggle with exercises such as overhead pressing or dumbbell shoulder raises, this routine can really help.

It's important never to push or force a stretch. The aim is to take the joint through its full end range of motion with control and without experiencing any pinching sensations. If you feel any pinching or sharp pains at a particular angle, just ease off a little and don't go too far into it. With any of these moves, the focus should be on control and moving your joints very slowly.

1

KNEELING LAT STRETCH

A. Start by kneeling on the floor. Place the fingertips or hands on the ground.

B. Keeping the arms as straight as possible, drive your fingers or hands down into the floor and lean back into your heels. As you do this, contract your abs to feel the lats stretch even more. Take a few deep breaths – and with each exhale, focus on relaxing the muscles and taking the stretch deeper. Rock back out of the stretch for a few seconds and repeat for 2 minutes.

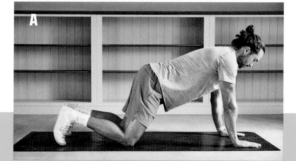

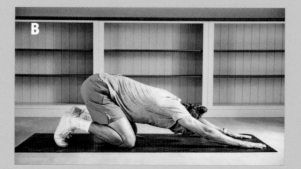

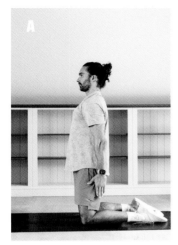
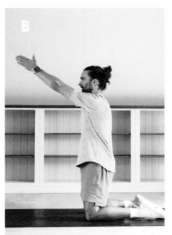
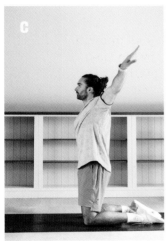
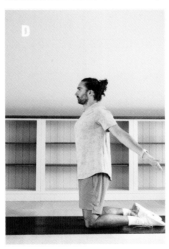

2

CONTROLLED SHOULDER ROTATIONS

A. Kneel down with both arms by your sides, palms facing the sides of your legs.

B. Keeping one arm as straight as possible and in that position, begin to raise the other arm up in front of you.

C. When the arm is directly above the head, start to slowly and fully rotate it in its socket, as if you are drawing a large circle, until the arm is back by your side with the palm facing away from your leg.

D. Slowly begin to unwind the arm in the opposite direction back to the starting point. Do these circular rotations 3 times on the first arm, then swap and repeat on the other side.

THIS IS A FANTASTIC STRETCH FOR THE LARGE MUSCLES IN YOUR BACK KNOWN AS THE LATS (LATISSIMUS DORSI).

3 SWIMMERS

A. Lie flat on your front on the floor. Engage your core muscles and raise both arms straight up above the head. With all your strength, lift the arms off the ground and start to rotate your shoulder joint.

B. Bring the hands towards your lower back in a breaststroke motion until your palms are facing up towards the sky.

C. When the hands meet at the lower back, rest for a couple of seconds and then reverse the move until your arms are back in the starting position. Repeat the movement slowly for 2 minutes.

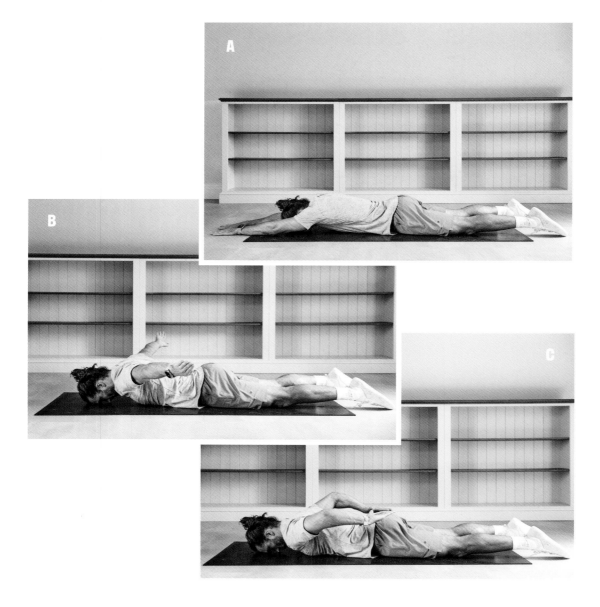

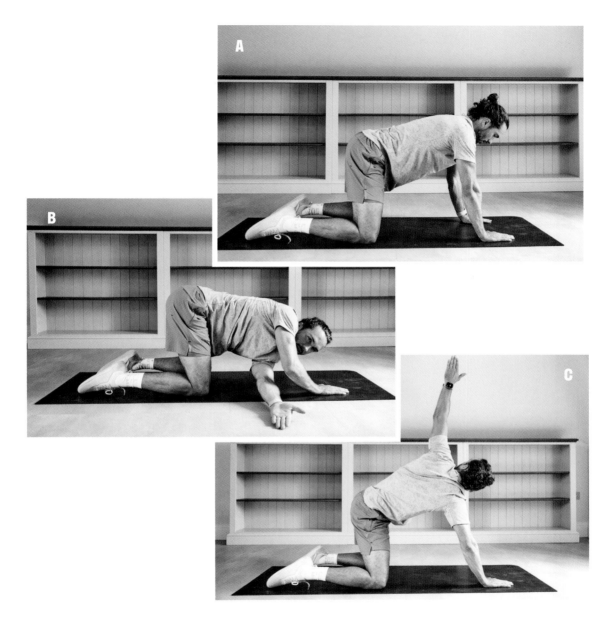

KNEELING REACH THROUGH TO T-OPEN

A. Kneel on all fours with your hands placed directly underneath your shoulders.

B. Take the left arm and thread it through the gap as far as you can to feel a stretch in your left shoulder.

C. Then slowly rotate at the spine and bring the left arm straight up over your head towards the sky. You'll feel a big stretch in the scapula as well as the pectoral muscles at the front. Do 1 minute of this on each arm.

5

STANDING ELBOW BUTTERFLIES

A. Standing straight, gently place the fingertips of both hands on the back of your head.

B. Slowly bring the elbows together until they touch. Then, using all of the muscles of your upper back and scapula, squeeze your elbows back towards the wall behind you. Repeat the movement very slowly for 2 minutes with big inhales and exhales.

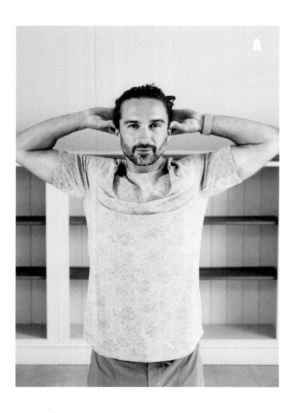

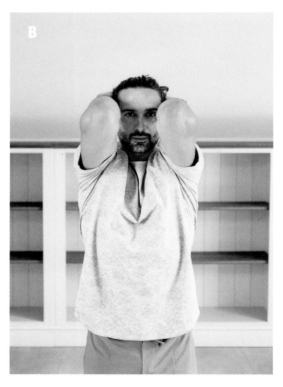

YOUR FOCUS SHOULD BE ON CONTROL AND MOVING YOUR JOINTS SLOWLY.

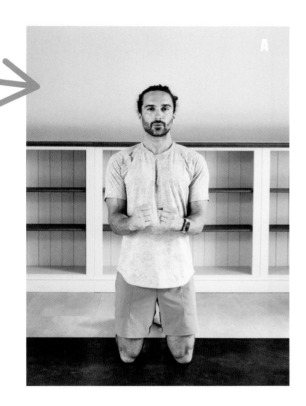

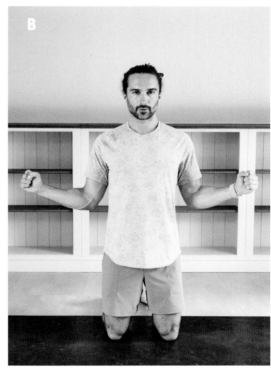

6

KNEELING SHOULDER EXTERNAL ROTATIONS

A. Start by kneeling on the floor. Bend your arms to 90 degrees and clench your fists.

B. Holding the angle, rotate your arms out towards your sides. Try to keep the elbows in contact with your torso and imagine you are stretching a large elastic band between your hands. Slowly bring the fists together and repeat for 2 minutes.

Please don't skip this chapter. I promise, it includes some really helpful advice. This section is all about those small daily wins and about how to reconnect with yourself and others. I have lots of simple but effective ways of boosting your mood or helping you feel that little bit calmer. There is something so rewarding about completing a little task, like when you tick off items on a to-do list. With every tick you build this sense of achievement, and it feels really motivating. Lots of the ideas and techniques in this chapter can be done with really low effort and input, so are great for those days when you just don't have the energy or mental capacity to exercise or do anything challenging. Remember there is no pressure to do all or any of these things everyday, but I truly believe every single time you manage to do any one of them you will feel better afterwards. Good luck. Have a wonderful day.

15-MINUTE HEALTH HACKS

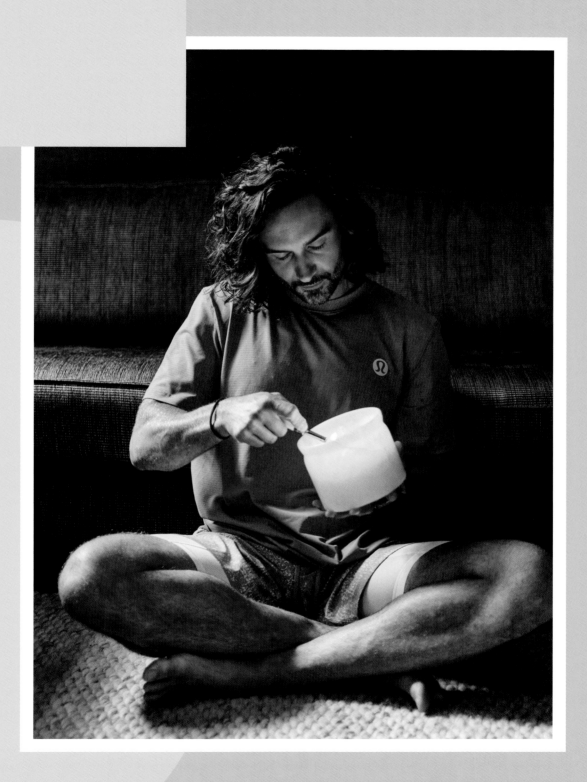

START YOUR DAY RIGHT

I think a good morning routine is vital when it comes to setting the tone for your day ahead. If you are someone who wakes up feeling stressed and tired after hitting the snooze button a few times and then ends up rushing to get to work, I have a few ideas for you to wake up feeling good and looking forward to the day ahead of you.

I know I bang on about sleep a lot, but the first step is to really commit to getting to bed a bit earlier and setting the intention the night before for what you want to achieve; see pages 216–221 for help on this.

If at all possible, I also really recommend starting your day with mindfulness (see page 228) or some morning exercise (see my 15-minute win below for inspiration). There are so many benefits to doing it first thing – firstly, it will energise you for the day and help remove any stress or anxiety you have about the day ahead. Secondly, it allows you to relax in the evening and socialise because you've already completed it and now have more free time after work.

It's very easy to wake up with a default negative mindset. Social media and the news really affects me, so I work hard on resisting the urge and instant impulse to check my phone as soon as I wake up. Delay it for as long as possible and focus on getting your mindset in a place of gratitude, and remember that life is beautiful. Everything will pass. Feel present. Shift your perspective.

And remember that your morning routine has to work for you. If you're suddenly finding yourself more stressed about missing parts of it than you were before you even had the routine, then it isn't working for you. So be adaptable and go with the flow – if you miss out sections of your routine, that's fine. You can take on the challenges. You can overcome anything that today throws at you. You've got this!

15 MINUTE WIN ←

Start this morning with 15 minutes of movement. It doesn't have to be intense. You could pick your favourite song and dance as you make breakfast. Or try this – step outside, set a quick timer for 7½ minutes and walk until the timer goes off, then turn around and walk back. Easy!

YOU'VE GOT THIS.

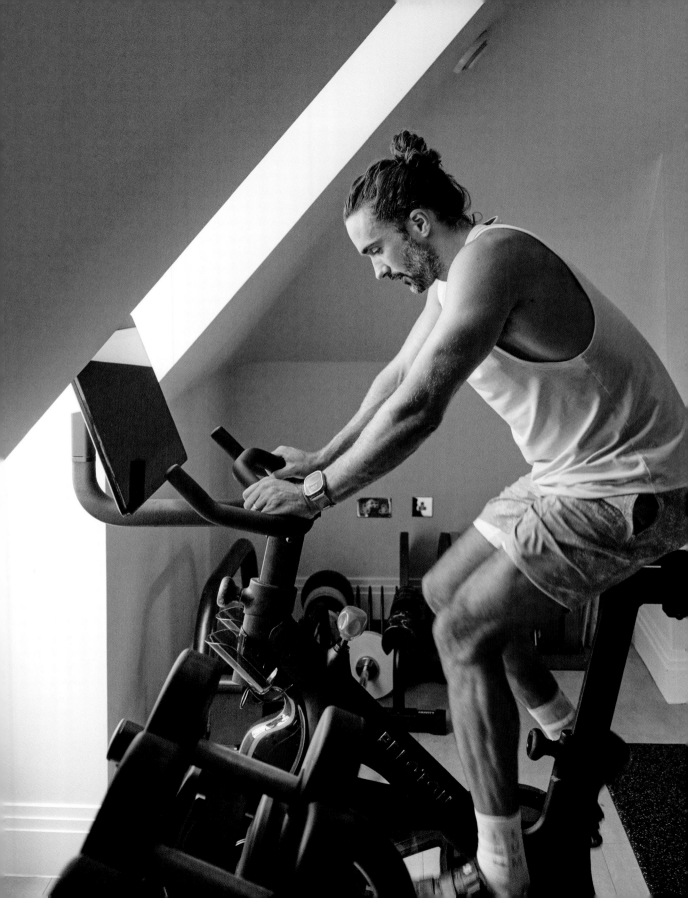

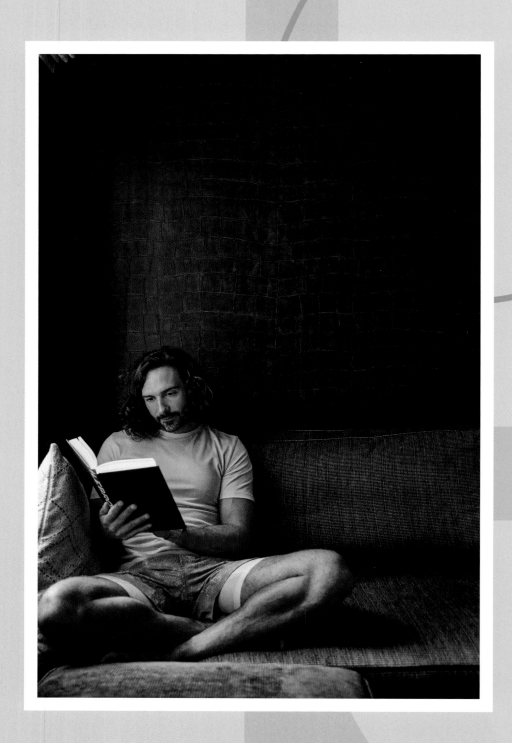

SLEEP

Sleep can be a hard thing to talk about. We all want more of it, but it's not always easy, especially if you have young children, work night shifts, experience insomnia, stress or anxiety, or if you are going through the menopause. So many things can get in the way of a good night's sleep and it can sometimes feel like it's out of our control. We do need to talk about it though, because sleep really is everything, and the more we understand how it impacts the body and mind, the better.

Sleep is the life force that fuels everything we do and something we must prioritise if we want to feel good physically and mentally. It is essential to every process in the human body, including muscle repair, hormone regulation, brain function and metabolism.

SLEEP SCIENCE

SLEEP IS ESSENTIAL

Being a parent to three children, I am more aware than ever of the impact of a lack of sleep can have on us all. In an ideal world, I would love to get 8 hours of deep, restorative, unbroken sleep each and every night, but with a teething baby going through a sleep regression we are often woken up multiple times during the night. This can also happen when we are stressed and anxious. This broken sleep means we wake up feeling sluggish and finding the motivation to do something that is good for our body becomes impossible. It makes the thought of exercising increasingly more difficult and I find that I end up eating a lot more sugary foods to try to pick up my energy levels.

Aside from these physical side effects, losing sleep can also have a massive impact on mood. If I'm tired, I inevitably wake up grumpy, feel way more impatient with the kids and am less motivated to cook, exercise, work or do anything even vaguely productive.

These feelings are a reminder that sleep affects so many areas of our lives and we really must prioritise it. It will give us balance, helps us feel good and allows us the energy to make better decisions each and every day. Think of good sleep as not optional, but essential.

I'm going to share my top tips and advice on what has helped me to get more sleep, and hopefully one of these will work for you too.

SLEEP 101

To better understand the importance of sleep, as well as the science behind it, I interviewed Dr Matthew Walker, the amazing sleep expert, on my podcast. I'm going to share some of those helpful insights with you here.

Sleep is essentially the foundation upon which everything else stands. Without adequate sleep, everything becomes more challenging.

I'm sure we have all experienced the dramatic drop in motivation and drive to exercise after we have a broken night's sleep. We also see a significant decrease in our willpower to eat healthy food when we are exhausted, and we often end up making poor choices and eating a lot more than usual. It's not just willpower at play though.

When we are sleep deprived, the levels of hormones (called leptin and ghrelin) that regulate our appetite can shift. We are more likely to be drawn to energy dense foods, and our brains are less effective at registering when we are full and satisfied by our meals. This is why the duration and quality of sleep is a huge factor in determining our body composition and is strongly linked to weight gain, which means that if weight loss is a goal of yours, then sleep should be your number one priority. Get that right and the rest will become much easier.

WHAT GOOD SLEEP CAN DO FOR YOU

There are so many benefits to good sleep, it really is the best change that you can make today. Whatever you can do to improve your quality of sleep is worth it. Here are just a few reasons to try to change your approach to how you rest:

BOOSTS YOUR MOOD

HELPS YOU TO MAINTAIN OR ACHIEVE A HEALTHY WEIGHT

IMPROVES CONCENTRATION

REDUCES ANXIETY AND RISK OF DEPRESSION

SUPPORTS YOUR IMMUNE SYSTEM

ENHANCES PHYSICAL ABILITY

ALLOWS YOU TO REGULATE YOUR EMOTIONS

15 MINUTE WIN

It's time to make a change. Keep it super-simple to start: go to bed 15 minutes earlier than you usually would. So if it's usually 11 p.m., try to make it so that you close your eyes at 10.45 p.m.

15 MINUTES TO A BETTER NIGHT'S SLEEP

TIP 1: HAVE A SET BED (AND WAKE-UP) TIME

We're always told that one of the best things we can do to improve the quality of our sleep is to go to bed and wake up at the same time every day. We as humans thrive off routine, and so does our sleep. So I decided to try it out. I chose times that worked for me (a bedtime of 10 p.m. and a wake-up time of 6 a.m.) and I fully committed to it. I did my best to stick to it every day, even on weekends (where possible!), and I can safely say it has had more of an impact on my health and fitness than anything else.

By prioritising sleep over watching TV or scrolling through reels until midnight, I find I am waking up with real energy and I feel motivated to do everything I want to get done in the day.

It has also completely reframed my thinking around sleep. Now I see an early night as an investment and not a sacrifice. This is something that really helps young children too. I often say we should create a culture of sleep in our homes and celebrate getting an early night. Everyone wakes up happier for it, and parenting feels a lot easier too. So start getting into a routine – pick a time to go to bed and to wake up and stick to it, even on weekends and holidays. If you need to adapt, try not to deviate from these times by more than an hour. Your body clock will thank you.

TIP 2: GET AN ALARM CLOCK

The easiest thing I've done to improve the quality of my sleep has been to invest in an alarm clock. It sounds so simple, but it's true. I got one of those illuminating sunrise alarm clocks, which mimics the sunrise to wake you up slowly and naturally, and plays soothing sounds like birds tweeting or waves rolling in to shore. It might not be for everyone, but I find it's such a pleasant way to wake up compared to the alarm on my phone, which I used to find so stressful and which I used to snooze time and time again.

But it's not just the sound that has made a difference. It's the fact that I'm not tempted to check my phone. Prior to getting an alarm clock, I relied solely on the alarm on my phone, which I kept on my bedside table. The same thing would happen all the time: I would wake up to go to the toilet, check the time on my phone without thinking and before I knew it I would be wide awake, sending DMs on Instagram, getting stressed out by news on Twitter or scrolling through random TikToks. It's such an unhealthy habit but it's so easy to get sucked into, and an hour can go past in the blink of an eye.

Investing in an alarm clock can have a huge impact, and I've never looked back. If it's not something you can get right now, another idea is to still set the alarm on your phone but leave it in the hallway outside your bedroom. This will help you to resist the urge to check your phone during the night, it will not allow you to hit snooze repeatedly and will hopefully help you to find that deeper, more restorative sleep that you are after.

(AND A HAPPIER MORNING)

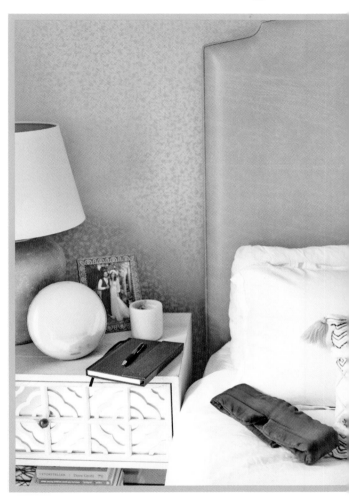

TIP 3: AVOID THE STRESS

So many things can cause us unnecessary stress and anxiety before bed. Sometimes we don't even realise we're doing it. This week, pay close attention to what you read, watch or listen to in the hours before you go to bed. Then ask yourself: is it helping you relax and unwind or is it filling your brain with stressful thoughts and worries?

If you like to read the news before bed but then find it hard to fall sleep because you've got one hundred negative, worrying things racing through your mind, try to avoid it – instead why not catch up on the news the following day during your lunch break?

If watching a true crime documentary is something you enjoy but you also find it stresses you out and makes you anxious before bed, try watching something funny, uplifting or calming instead, and save the more intense TV shows or films for an afternoon on the weekend.

These are small changes to your routine, but they can genuinely make a meaningful difference. Remember: every extra minute of sleep is a win.

15 MINUTE WIN

Take a look at your bedroom setup. Tidy your nightstand and make sure to have only the essentials on there – including your alarm clock. Make sure it feels like a welcoming and calming space. Try to keep the room as uncluttered as you can and keep everything you need for a good night's sleep to hand.

TIP 4: DITCH YOUR PHONE

This was hard for me to begin with because I was just so conditioned to be on my phone until the very last moment before I went to sleep. And as soon as the alarm went off in the morning, I'd pick up my phone, open my social media apps – and boom, within two seconds I'd be plugged into the algorithm and giving myself no chance to breathe and feel present in a new day.

This is something we have to get a hold on. It's about learning to set boundaries, detach from your phone and win back some hours in the day. All we can do is try to make some small changes to limit our use and reduce our average daily screen time and pick-ups.

I find that by not having the phone in the bedroom I have more time for reading to my children and for communicating with my wife, Rosie, at the end of the day. Nothing is more important or urgent than being present and giving my family my full attention. It allows me to fall asleep more easily and feel much calmer in the morning because I'm not instantly in a state of stress or anger from being triggered by something online. It gives me time to feel present, to think, to feel grateful or to plan ideas for the day ahead. The 15 minutes without my phone when I wake up flies by and usually involves all the normal things that would usually start your day – going to the bathroom, brushing my teeth, showering (I recommend a cold one, see page 235!) and getting dressed.

It is important to remember that you will not achieve this every day, especially immediately when you are trying so hard to break a conditioned habit. Even as I write this, I still struggle with consistently leaving my phone out of the bedroom or not looking at my social media the split second I wake up. Just keep challenging that urge and temptation to go online straight away and remind yourself how much better your mind feels when you have that first part of the day or last part of the day screen-free and calm.

THIS IS ABOUT LEARNING TO SET GOOD BOUNDARIES. DETACH YOURSELF FROM YOUR PHONE AND WIN BACK SOME POSITIVE FEELINGS AND A FEW EXTRA HOURS IN THE DAY.

15 MINUTE WIN

Set yourself the daily goal of not looking at your phone for the first 15 minutes when you wake up in the morning. This will be really tough at first, and you won't always achieve it; even I struggle. But always keep going, because it does get easier – and when you do get that little break in the morning, it will feel incredible.

TIP 5: WIND DOWN WITH A BOOK BEFORE BED

Once you start to reduce your screen time, it's a good idea to replace the habit with one that helps you wind down and relax into sleep. It's important to have a bedtime routine, so that your brain and body recognises when it's time to start winding down. Change into your pyjamas, dim the lights, write in your journal – whatever helps you slow down and get ready for bed. This will look different for everyone.

One thing that is really effective is just reading a good old-fashioned book, either alone in bed to help you nod off or with your children. Reading stories together is a wonderful way of bonding with your kids and it has been proven to be hugely beneficial for both them and you. It also releases the 'love' hormone oxytocin, which helps ease you into sleep with a peaceful state of mind. Reading with children has lots of great benefits – it can help improve your children's empathy, increase vocabulary and improve emotional regulation. It is one of my favourite things in the world to do, and I'll be honest I now read more with my kids than I ever would do on my own.

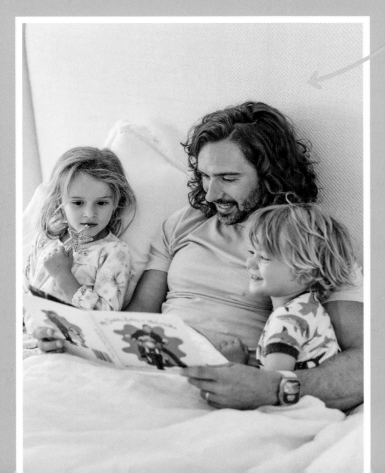

15 MINUTE WIN

Aim for at least 15 minutes of reading a day. Again, that doesn't always happen and that's OK. Start with just 5 or 10 minutes a day, and start to build the time. As I say, any reading time is meaningful and beneficial, so just experiment and find what works for you and what works for your family; it is well worth persevering with to make it part of your small daily wins.

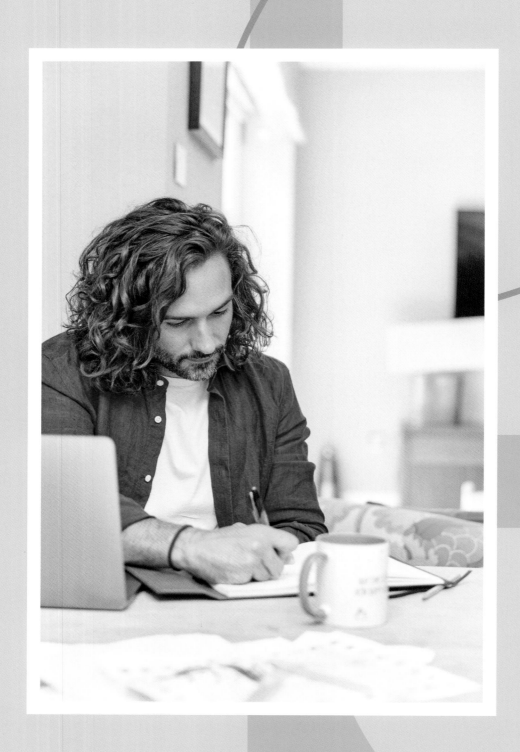

YOUR MIND

Having a positive mindset and looking after our mental health is so important. There is so much pressure coming at us from every direction. Social media is constantly telling us to do more, to hustle, to be the very best versions of ourselves that we can be. It's a lot. That's why I've put together some techniques you can turn to if you ever feel you need a boost – from journaling and practising gratitude to mindfulness and listening to podcasts, to the power of cold-water therapy (yes, there will be ice baths).

I've shown you how to nourish your body; now I want to show you how to feel good and nourish your mind. It's not always easy to do this stuff, especially if you're feeling down or stressed or overwhelmed, but in just as little as 15 minutes you can start to change how you feel. It won't happen overnight, but over time small changes can lead to big results. Start small and build from there.

JOURNALING

Journaling has been shown to be a powerful tool and a brilliant coping strategy for supporting our mental health. It can help you prioritise your problems, fears and concerns. You can track any symptoms day-to-day, so that you can recognise triggers and learn ways to better control them. Writing things down on paper provides an opportunity for letting go of negative thoughts and practising positive self-talk. Other benefits include:

REDUCING ANXIETY

BREAKING CYCLES OF OBSESSIVE THINKING AND BROODING

IMPROVING OUR AWARENESS AND PERCEPTION OF EVENTS

REGULATING EMOTIONS

BOOSTING PHYSICAL HEALTH

Why not give it a try? Some of the best times to journal are as soon as you wake up in the morning or just before bed. Make it easy for yourself – put your journal where you will see it, like on your bedside table for as soon as you wake up (instead of reaching for your phone, reach for your journal!) or with your coffee cup in the kitchen. The most important thing is to set aside some dedicated time and that way build it into your routine.

People often ask me what they should write. I know it can be very hard when you've got a blank page in front of you. The number one thing to remember is that there is no right or wrong way to journal. You can write whatever comes into your head, make lists or use writing prompts. You can get down your thoughts, worries or fears, you can brainstorm your goals or you can come up with some positive affirmations. You can even doodle if it helps.

HOW TO NOURISH YOUR MIND

Nine times out of ten, if I have to choose between journaling and exercise, I will turn to exercise. That's just what works best for me. It's how I process and release what's going on inside my head. But keeping a journal is another incredibly powerful outlet; it's been proven to work wonders and it might work best for you. The key is to try different things and see what daily changes feel good. Imagine how much better you would feel if today you dedicated 15 minutes to journaling instead of scrolling on Instagram.

15 MINUTE WIN

Grab your journal and a pen and sit in a comfortable position. Start writing for 15 minutes. Here are a few helpful prompts:

☐ **What has your day been like, and why?**

☐ **Where are you happiest? Describe that place.**

☐ **When you can't fall asleep, what's on your mind?**

☐ **What is important to you right now?**

☐ **Where do you want to be in five years?**

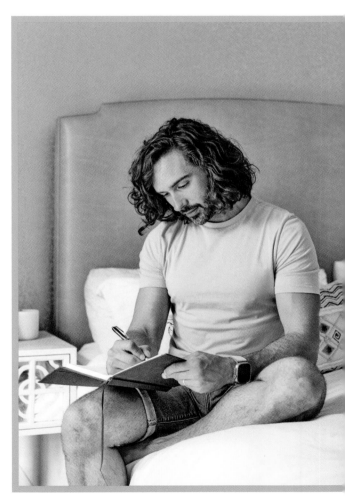

GRATITUDE

What is gratitude and what does it really mean to feel grateful? Gratitude is a positive feeling we get when we focus on what's good in our lives and we are thankful for the things we have. It's about pausing for a moment to notice and appreciate the things we often take for granted, like having a roof over our heads, food in the fridge and clean water running from the taps, as well as our health and the friends and family who love us. It's not always easy to find a sense of gratitude, especially if you are feeling down, stressed, anxious or overwhelmed, but trust me: it's really worth it.

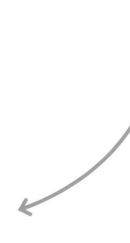

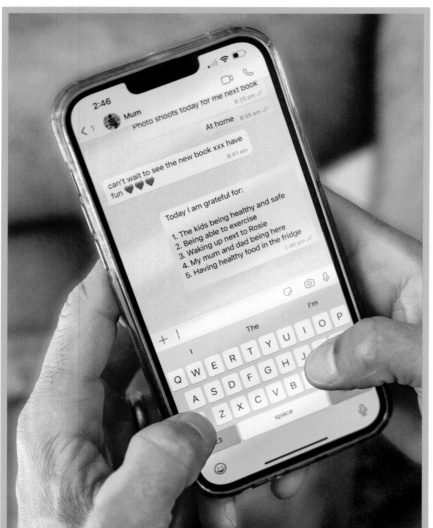

Practising gratitude can help you refocus and anchor yourself in the present moment. A great way to do this is through gratitude journaling. This is about taking the practice of journaling and focusing on writing only about the things that bring you joy and that you want to recognise you're grateful for.

Take a minute to write down some good things that happened today or something you're excited about. It doesn't need to be a full-on diary entry with paragraphs of text; it could be just three short bullet points. It might be as simple as writing down one thing that made you smile.

IF YOU'RE STUCK, HERE ARE THREE PROMPTS TO HELP YOU GET STARTED:

1 I am grateful for who I am because…

2 I am grateful for my family because…

3 Something silly that I am grateful for is…

WHATSAPP GRATITUDE

I don't manage to write in a diary or journal very often because I find I get too easily distracted. Instead, I practise gratitude in a much simpler way: using WhatsApp. First, I usually write down 3–5 things I feel grateful for that day. For example, 'I am grateful to wake up in a warm house with my children safe' or 'I am grateful for my mum still being in my life' or 'I am grateful to have a wife who loves me'. I then forward these points separately to the important people in my life. The reason for doing this is to voice the things I feel lucky and thankful to have, and by sharing it with my loved ones those bullet points go from being a thought in my head to a conscious feeling.

WANT TO TRY IT? YOU COULD START YOUR MESSAGE WITH:

☐ Thank you for being…

☐ What I love most about you is…

☐ I had the best time when we…

The intention behind sharing what I'm grateful for isn't to get a list of things sent back to me in return, but that is what almost always happens. It feels so good because then you all go about your day with smiles on your faces, thinking about the things that mean the most to you.

15 MINUTE WIN

Set aside 15 minutes today to sit down with a piece of paper or the notes app on your phone and jot down a couple of things you're grateful for. If you feel comfortable, maybe even share it with the people that you mention. You might be surprised how good you can feel after doing something so simple.

MINDFULNESS

When we think of mindfulness, the first thing we often think about is meditation. If meditation isn't something you've tried before, a great place to start is with apps like Headspace or Calm, or by simply searching for 'guided meditations' on YouTube. There are so many great guided meditations that focus on dealing with different feelings and emotions, such as anxiety, fear or grief.

But mindfulness can actually be achieved in many different ways. I'll be honest, I've tried meditation many times. I think it's amazing and I do feel the benefits of it, but no matter how much I force myself to try to keep it up, it doesn't seem to stick as a regular habit. Instead, I've had to find other ways to be mindful. Mindfulness is all about finding an activity that slows down your mind and helps you to focus, connect with your breath and feel a sense of calm. There are actually many simple methods in life for how to do this.

Find activities that help you slow down, connect with your breath and bring you a sense of calm. These will be really helpful on days when you need to settle your mind. You might find that doing some gentle stretching or yoga really helps to centre you and bring you back to your equilibrium. My number one piece of advice? Find what works for you. Mindfulness looks different for everyone, and that's OK.

The things that work for me are:

GOING FOR WALKS IN NATURE

STRETCHING

COLOURING WITH THE KIDS

WATERING THE PLANTS

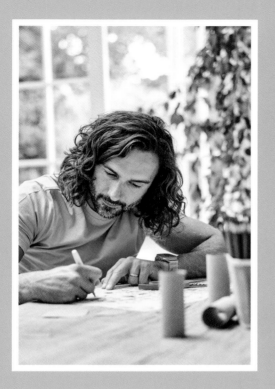

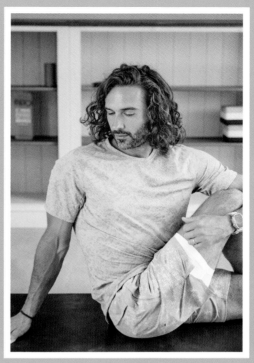

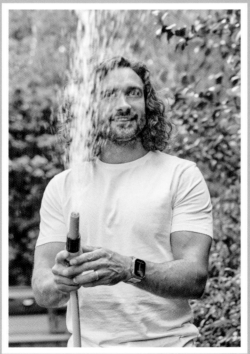

15 MINUTE WIN ←

If you're feeling stressed or overwhelmed, try 15 minutes of mindfulness right now. Going for a 'mindfulness walk' is a great place to start, especially if you're not a big fan of sitting still. Just pop out for a stroll and make an extra effort to look around and take in your surroundings. Something as simple as this can really help put you in a more positive frame of mind.

MUSIC FOR EVERY MOOD

Music is transformative. It has the power to make you laugh or cry or feel a sense of calm, and it is another wonderful tool to use when feeling stressed or anxious. I personally use music a lot to help me get through the day and put me in a certain mood. I use it to hype myself up for a workout or to wind down after a busy day.

MIXTAPE

Here are some of the artists and bands I like to listen to, whether I'm looking for a pick-me-up or simply to relax:

MUSIC AS MEDITATION

Music is brilliant when it comes to mindfulness. It can provide a calming backdrop for meditation, and you can also use it to practise being in the present moment, through what's called 'active listening'. This means focusing solely on the music that you re listening to, and ignoring anything else going on around you. I think it's almost impossible to feel stressed when listening to certain songs. Invest some time into finding out what music makes you feel a certain way and then make a conscious decision to utilise its power to change how you feel today. You can even take this one step further and learn how to play an instrument. Learning a new skill is a brilliant way to focus your mind and improve your mood, and you will find you cannot think about anything else.

→ **WORK OUT:** I listen to Eminem and Arctic Monkeys when I work out to get pumped and focused.

→ **RELAX:** I listen to Ludovico Einaudi and Max Richter when I'm feeling stressed and want to feel calm.

→ **CHILL WITH THE KIDS:** I listen to chilled jazz music or lullaby playlists when I'm cooking and eating with the kids.

→ **BOOST YOUR MOOD:** I listen to Bob Marley and the Wailers when I'm making breakfast or cleaning the dishes, because it always makes me happy and puts me in a good mood.

15 MINUTE WIN

Take 15 minutes to actively listen to some music. It's really simple. Put on a calming album or playlist (I recommend Ludovico Einaudi's music; it is magical), get comfortable and close your eyes. Take some big, deep breaths and take a few minutes to do nothing except focus on the piece of music. That means no texting, no reading, no scrolling: all of your attention goes into listening.

YOU CAN EVEN TAKE THIS ONE STEP FURTHER AND LEARN HOW TO PLAY AN INSTRUMENT. LEARNING A NEW SKILL IS A BRILLIANT WAY TO FOCUS YOUR MIND AND IMPROVE YOUR MOOD, AS YOU WILL FIND YOU CANNOT THINK ABOUT ANYTHING ELSE WHILE TRYING TO PICK UP THIS NEW SKILL.

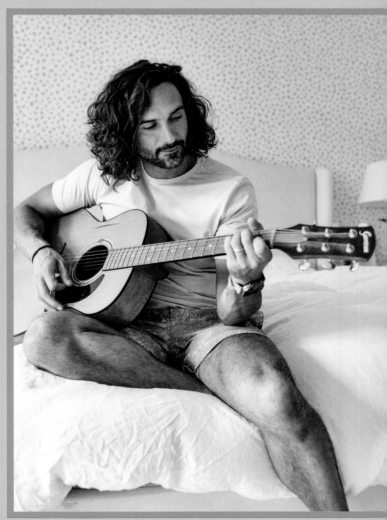

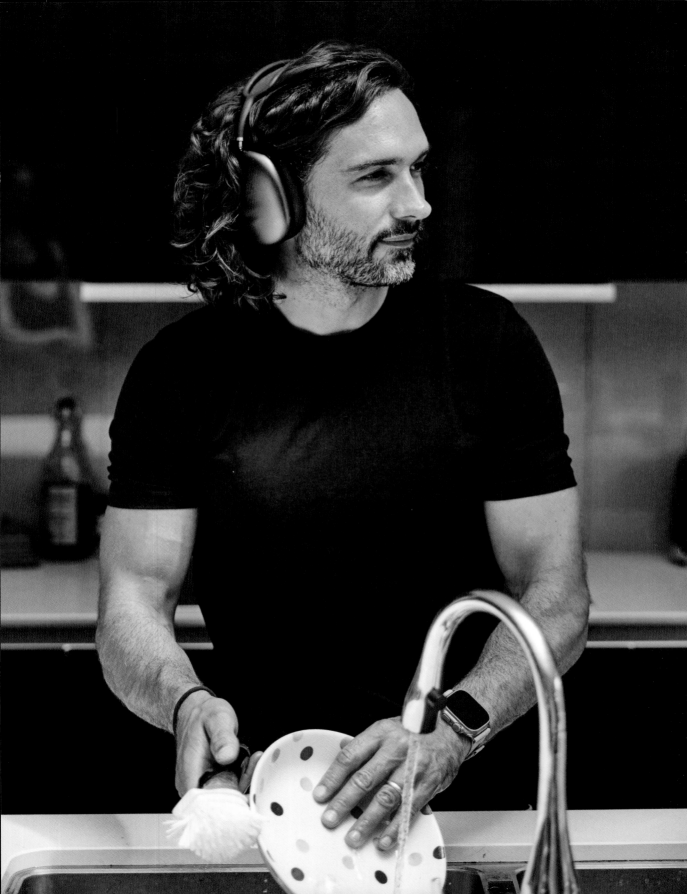

PODCASTS TO FEEL GOOD

I'm a big fan of podcasts. I think they are a great way to learn and absorb information. There are so many genres out there now, too. I think it's important to listen to conversations that put you in a good mood or help you to learn something new rather than cause you to feel stressed or anxious.

There are plenty of podcasts that are uplifting and designed to help listeners feel calm, inspired and motivated. Two of my favourite podcasts are 'Happy Place' by Fearne Cotton and 'How I Built This' by Guy Raz. They always feature interesting conversations with good people trying to share a positive message. Some other great motivational and self-help podcasts are 'How To Fail', 'On Purpose with Jay Shetty' and 'Happier with Gretchen Rubin'.

PODCASTS AND MOTIVATION

Podcasts are a brilliant tool to utilise when training. I have friends who train for long-distance races and swear by podcasts and audiobooks. Music can get repetitive, especially if you are running for an hour or more. And if you get a good enough podcast, it encourages you to keep going to hear to the end (or that's the hope at least!). I have a friend who will only listen to their favourite podcast on a run – so they have to run if they want to hear the latest episode. Tough love, but it works!

A lot of people say that podcasts also help them to feel less alone. The people chatting and laughing in your ear keep you company – a bit like how your gran used to have the radio playing in the background.

I have learned so much from podcasts – both listening to them and making my own. You get to speak to and hear from the most fascinating people, people you might never encounter otherwise. You get to listen in on really interesting conversations between people with perspectives that are different to your own. It's a way to connect with people and stories and broaden your horizons. So look for podcasts that help you become the best version of yourself and take a listen.

→ **15 MINUTE WIN**

Podcasts are great for motivating you to do things you don't want to. For me, it's chores. I find I like to listen to podcasts when I do the dishes. It helps to distract me from the task at hand and make the time pass a lot quicker.

COLD-WATER THERAPY

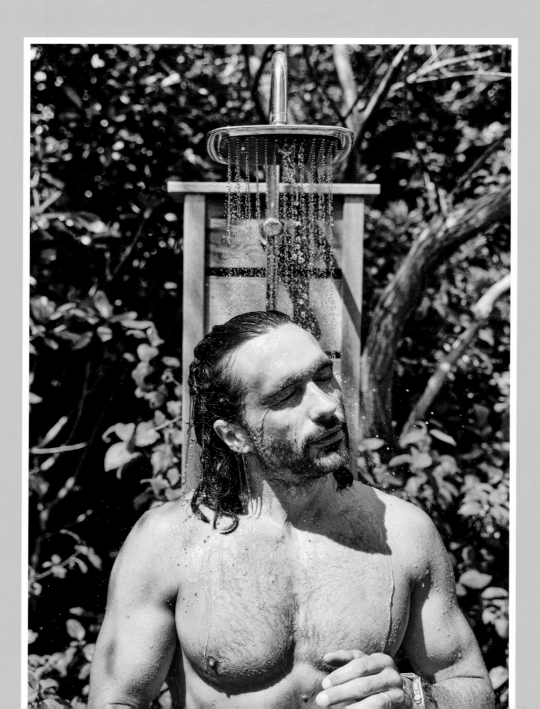

Cold showers? Ice baths? Are you mad? Maybe a little bit, but there is a load of research and science to back up the method behind the madness that is immersing yourself in cold water. You may have heard about Wim Hof, also known as The Iceman, who has been talking about the physical and mental benefits of ice-cold water for decades. Though it's not a new phenomenon, cold-water therapy has grown in popularity recently, mainly through social media. You often see someone on Instagram or TikTok jumping into a bath full of ice, cutting a hole in a frozen lake in Norway or standing under a cold running shower. It seems that more and more people are getting curious and going on a quest to experience the benefits of cold water.

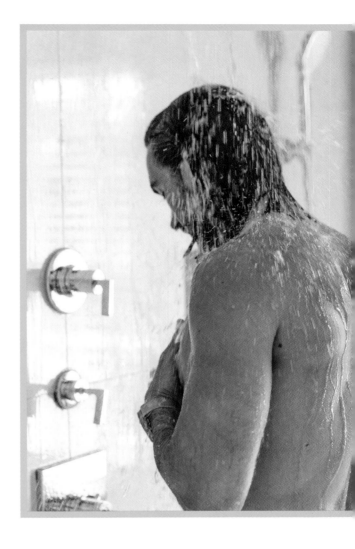

COLD SHOWERS

Cold-water therapy may sound like your idea of hell, but believe me, it really is incredible. I started out by doing a 7-day cold shower challenge at home. Every morning for a week, I took a cold shower for just 30 seconds. I went with the cold in and cold out approach. That meant no warm running water at all. You might prefer to start with a warm shower and end with the last 30 seconds on cold. There is no right or wrong way to do it; I just find the instant hit of cold invigorates me more and the dopamine hit feels more potent.

BREATHE LIKE A BOSS

Breathing is everything when it comes to cold-water therapy. When the cold water first hits you, you will find yourself taking shallow, rapid breaths, and sometimes you will hold your breath. The best piece of advice I can give you is to take a big exhale right before you step into the cold shower or ice bath. This means that the first breath you are forced to take is an inhale. The goal from then on is to focus on taking slow, controlled deep breaths. This will help you to feel calm and overcome the inevitable urge to scream and jump straight out…

ICE BATHS

I used to hate feeling cold but over time I have become more comfortable with being uncomfortable. I no longer fear or dread it – I actually embrace it and chase the colder temperatures. The initial cold short showers led me to the next step: the ice bath, or taking a short dip in very cold water.

Ice baths have so many benefits. They can help to boost your central nervous system, reduce inflammation in the body and decrease muscle soreness. Research shows that cold water stimulates the vagus nerve (part of the parasympathetic nervous system), which drops your blood pressure and pulse. Not only that, a hormone called norepinephrine is released in your brain with cold exposure, which can increase endorphin production.

IMPORTANT NOTE

Ice baths can be a lot of fun, but they're absolutely not for everyone. They are not advised if you have a pre-existing cardiovascular disease, high blood pressure or type 1 or type 2 diabetes. If for any reason you suspect you should give the ice bath a miss or are in any way anxious, please always speak to your doctor first.

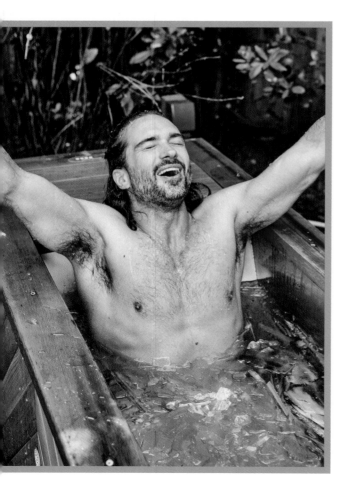

HOW TO DO IT

I'm really lucky that my bath generates its own ice, but you can easily create an ice bath at home too. All you need to do is grab a few large bags of ice from the supermarket and throw them in the bathtub along with some cold water. Anything under 10°C is considered beneficial. A great hack is to make your own mini icebergs. I do this by filling large Tupperware containers with water and sticking them in the freezer. Just 3 or 4 of them can really help lower the temperature. And don't worry, you don't have to stay in for too long. I usually aim for around 1–3 minutes at a time.

15 MINUTE WIN

Set yourself a cold-water challenge this week. You don't even need 15 minutes to do this one – it could mean flashing on the cold water at the end of your morning shower or carving out 1 minute on a Sunday to try your very first ice bath. You might be surprised by just how good you will feel in your body and mind. Good luck!

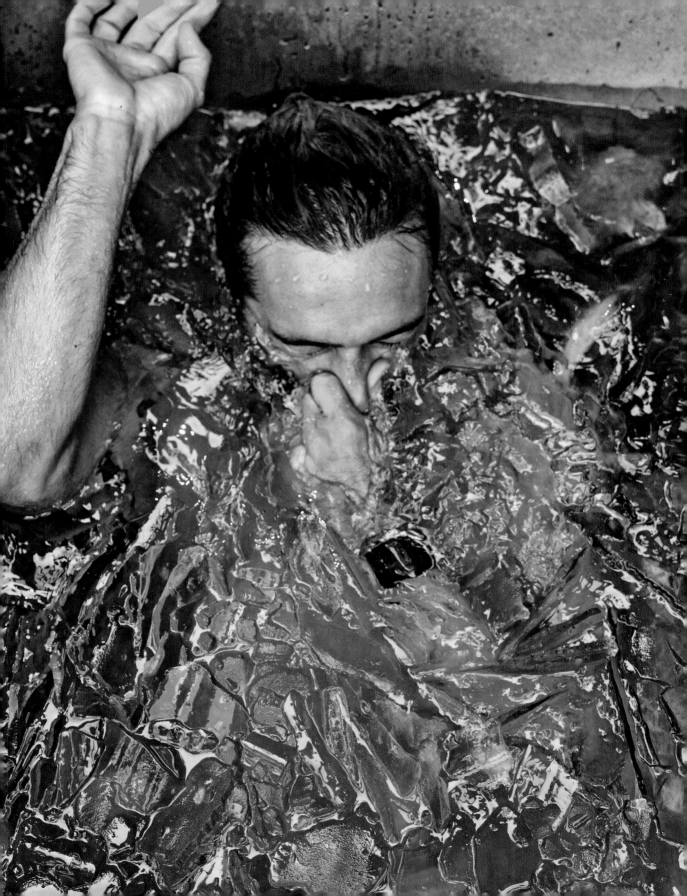

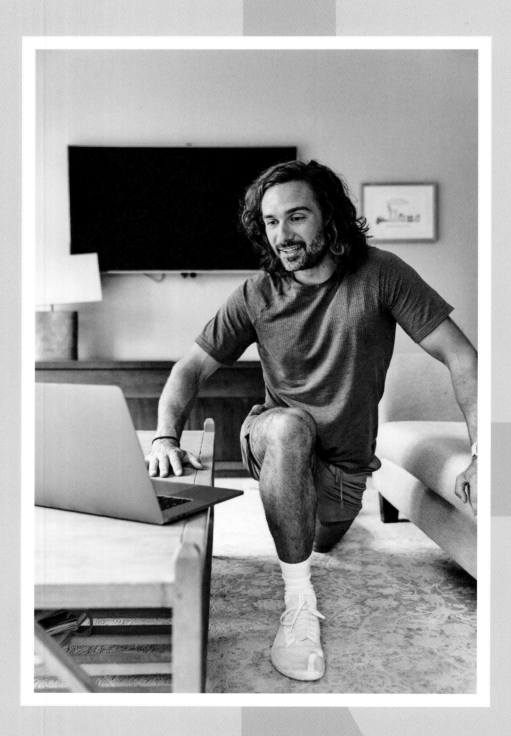

LIFESTYLE

It is so hard to balance everything. Sometimes just getting to the end of the week can feel like an uphill struggle. That's why I wanted to write about two of the most important things in a lot of our lives: work and relationships. Work takes up so much of our time, and it's way too easy to let it take over. I want to show you how you can take back control and as much as possible be in charge of your own day. I've got some simple but effective suggestions to help you shake things up and reprioritise, and I also want to give you strategies so that when you do have to produce the goods, you can focus on the task in front of you 100%.

At the end of the day it's so important to learn how to set boundaries and find a better work/life balance. That way you can then have more time (and more energy) to do what matters most to you; for me, that's spending time with Rosie and the kids. Because really it's all about doing what you enjoy with the people you care about, whether that's your partner, friends and family, or your kids.

ADDRESSING WORK/LIFE BALANCE

Something we all strive for is a good work/life balance. This is not always easy to achieve, especially if you have young children and a busy career, but it's so important to be aware of how to avoid burnout and stress. Stress is something which accumulates over time and builds up in the body. This will have an impact on your mental health, but the effects of long-term pressure and stress can be physical too. Stress and physical exhaustion can cause fatigue, digestive issues, skin rashes, high blood pressure, muscle aches, headaches and much more, so this is something we must take seriously and always challenge. Here I've included some ideas for how to strike a balance, but if you are worried then do reach out to your doctor.

FINISH UP ON TIME

A real crunch point is finishing work on time. We've all experienced 'the creep' and how easy it is to continue working in the evening. But you need to take this time back for yourself. If you don't do it, no one else will. So decide a reasonable cut-off point. Say to yourself that at 6 p.m. sharp you will stand up from the desk. Do whatever you need to do to make yourself step away – schedule an appointment, book an exercise class or arrange to meet a friend after work.

15 MINUTE WIN

One of the first things that always slips is taking your lunch break and therefore nourishment. It's so easy when you're working to cobble together a sandwich and sit back down at your desk, or to forget about lunch altogether. But this is your time – start by taking back 15 minutes for yourself. For 15 minutes, sit outside, go for a walk around the block, call your mum. Time away from the screen will make you more productive in the long run, and 15 minutes of fresh air and Vitamin D will beat staring at your inbox any day.

UNPLUG

15-MINUTE HEALTH HACKS LIFESTYLE

It's so common for people to feel pressure to be available and online all of the time. With more people working from home or working a hybrid model between office and home, the lines between the two are now blurred. It's important to set boundaries with work and prioritise downtime. To allow yourself time to unplug, switch off and be unreachable. When you finish work for the day, you need to be able to rest. Make it clear to your employer (or to yourself if you are the boss) that certain hours during the evening and weekends are not for work. Turn off your devices if you can or turn off all notifications and add an out-of-office response on your email. By setting these clear boundaries, you manage everyone's expectations and reduce the pressure on yourself. You can then find more time for the balance side of things by having more time to relax, exercise or socialise.

The key takeaway is this: the more balance you achieve, the better you will feel, and the more productive you will be when you do sit down to work. When you're off, be off. Don't check your emails after hours or on weekends, and physically put your laptop and/or work phone away when you're not working. Work will always be there. There will always be more emails. Being productive feels great, but it's also fundamentally important that we look after ourselves too.

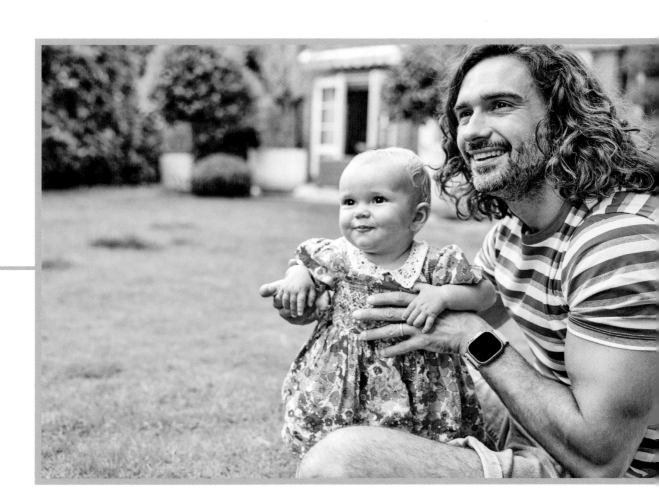

DROP
EVERYTHING
AND FOCUS

I am going to be completely honest: I find it really hard to concentrate. I struggle to focus on any task for long periods of time without getting distracted. In fact, even right now as I write this chapter, I find myself constantly picking up my phone trying to stimulate my mind and get a hit of dopamine. I am working on it though, and one way I have managed to start improving my focus is by challenging myself and almost gamifying my focus and attention to help me stay on task.

I do this by putting my phone next to me open with the stopwatch running. The aim and intention is to complete 15 minutes of focused work with zero distraction. No podcast. No music. No pick-ups.

At first, I found this almost impossible, and through habit and a desire to procrastinate or distract myself, I literally found myself checking the stopwatch and picking up my phone within 2–3 minutes. What's remarkable though is the sense of achievement when I actually get to 15 minutes, knowing I have been on task and that I have been able to concentrate. It feels so good because it's my brain rewarding my efforts and giving me a little dopamine. Fifteen minutes is a great place to start, too, because research shows it takes around 15 minutes to get into a flow state where ideas come and concentration increases.

Soon 15 minutes doesn't seem that hard, and before you know it, you are determined and motivated to do even longer, then 30 minutes goes by and you've still not picked up your phone to check your favourite apps. Success!

15 MINUTE WIN

Give this a try next time you want to stay focused on a task. It could be writing in your diary, replying to emails, reading a book or even doing the housework or organising your wardrobe. Set a timer for 15 minutes, put your phone down and concentrate on the task at hand and nothing else. It feels really good to get small tasks done, and the more you practise, the better you will get.

WALKING AND TALKING

One of the most positive things we have implemented as part of the Body Coach team is something I like to call 'walkie talkies'. This is when you have a call which doesn't require you to see someone on video or share a screen. Instead of sitting at your desk, you use the time to take the call on the move.

It's such a huge win in so many ways. You'll be amazed at how productive these walks and talks can be for yourself and your team. Not only will you be getting outside in the fresh air and getting your daily steps in, you'll also be more energised, more focused and have much better ideas. Being outside in nature also stimulates your creativity and helps you to feel calmer and less stressed.

I often see members of the team go out on 5- and 10-kilometre walkie talkies and they always stroll back into the office with smiles on their faces and so much more energy. This is something which isn't unrealistic and can be incorporated into your day. I really encourage all companies to give it a try.

15 MINUTE WIN

This doesn't need to be in a work context either. Next time there's a friend or family member you want to call and have a catch up with, try doing a walkie talkie with them. You are literally winning every time you get out and get those steps in.

IT TAKES AROUND 15 MINUTES TO GET INTO A FLOW STATE WHERE IDEAS COME AND CONCENTRATION INCREASES.

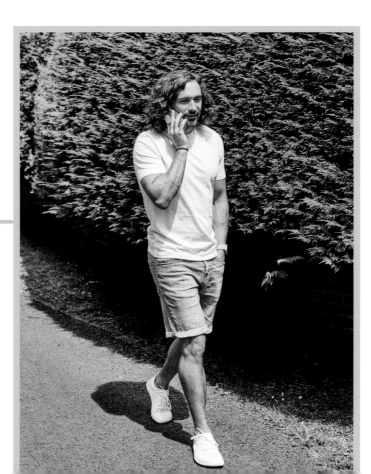

VALUING YOUR PARTNER

One thing I believe is really important for a happy and healthy relationship is valuing, respecting and appreciating your partner. It's really easy to focus on what we do in a relationship and the stress and pressures we experience every day. We can get tunnel vision and forget to think about the other person's feelings or responsibilities. But it's so important to zoom out and think about the contribution your partner makes towards your life and acknowledge all the things that they do.

SHOW THEM YOU CARE

A nice idea is to spend 15 minutes writing down all the small and big tasks your partner does in a week or month for you and your family. You might think the list of things they do is bigger or smaller than yours and that's OK, but then imagine if you had to do all of those things yourself on top of your current responsibilities. You can then quickly start to feel grateful for just how important that person is in your life and how you are a team. You are here to support each other. This can also highlight ways that you can help to support each other and tasks you might share.

If you find it hard sitting down and saying you love and appreciate your partner to their face, why not write a letter for them at work or send a voice note for them to listen to on the way home? A simple text saying: 'I know it's stressful. Thank you for getting the kids to school on time this week. You are an amazing parent' or 'I really appreciate you working hard this week and providing us with a fridge full of food' can put such a big smile on someone's face. Not only will your partner feel happy and loved, it will also make you feel good because being kind and giving love always feels good.

15 MINUTE WIN

Spend 15 minutes writing down all the things you love about your partner. It can refocus your appreciation and love for them, and it is really important to verbalise this, so do share this list with them when you are done.

CARVE OUT SOME QUALITY TIME TOGETHER

Another thing that I think is super-important for a relationship is prioritising time alone to talk without anyone else around. This is obviously much more challenging when you have young kids, but even if you can't manage a date night outside of the house it is still possible to find 15 minutes alone together before bed. Catching up on the day and what's going on in someone else's life is really important. Listening and letting each other vent or get something off your chest is always a positive thing and helps them (and you) to feel fully supported.

It's also really powerful to talk about your goals and dreams for the future. This can help you both realign and remember why you are in this together and have chosen to spend your lives together. Talking and planning for the future brings you closer. You will feel heard and understood and this will help you to fall asleep and wake up a little bit calmer and happier.

So make time for each other. In the same way feeling grateful about something makes you feel good, telling someone else you are grateful for them can really help them feel valued and appreciated too, and as humans we all need and want to feel that.

15 MINUTE WIN

Switch the TV off early this evening and make 15 minutes of time for each other to catch up on the highlights of your day and any problems you are facing. As they say, a problem shared is a problem halved.

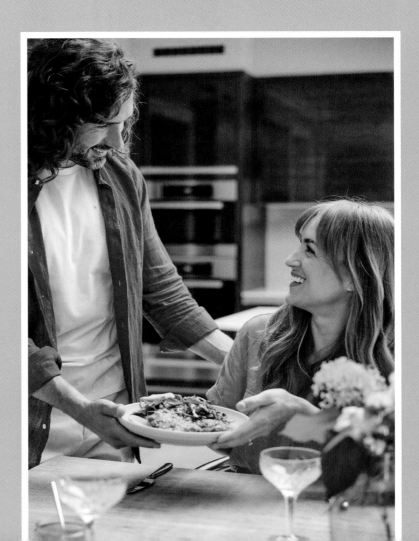

HAVING FUN AS A FAMILY

In today's fast-moving digital world, it's very easy to spend a huge part of each day looking at screens. I'm a big fan of doing non-screen activities together as a family. Just old-school, pre-iPad and phone stuff. Stepping away from our devices is not only important for our mental health, it can really improve communication and connection with our children.

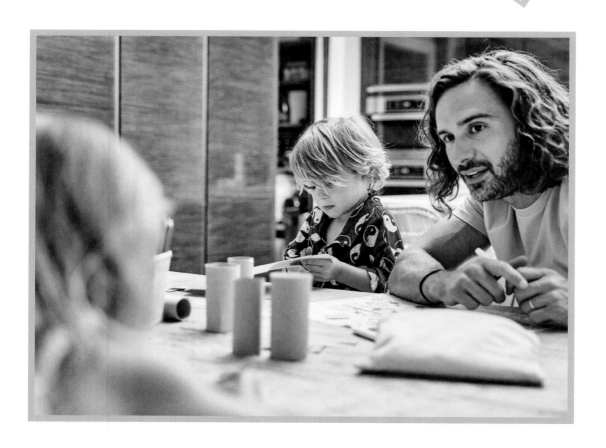

GET CREATIVE

We love doing creative activities like arts and crafts, such as making a birthday card, colouring in a picture book or finding stones from the garden and painting them. These calming activities can really help to release stress and tension from your body and can help you feel that closer bond with your children. Two other really fun activities we have got into lately with the kids are the card games Uno and Dobble. These are great entertainment alternatives to screen time when eating out or when travelling together. We always make sure we take them in our bag when we go out and the kids really love playing them with us.

GO OUTSIDE

As a family, we also try to get as much time outside as possible away from screens and devices. Even on colder days, we find that our children are much happier being outside as long as we wrap up warm. Nature really is medicine and it's healing in so many ways. Sunlight helps increase the brain's release of a hormone called serotonin, which has mood-boosting effects and can help you feel calm and focused. Another wonderful benefit of nature and sunlight is that it really helps with getting a good night's sleep. Whenever possible, we love to do fun and energetic activities outside, like hide-and-seek, climbing trees, playing basketball or riding our bikes or scooters around the block.

These suggestions are about creating moments of interaction, talking, laughing and connecting which makes you all feel a little bit happier. I hope some of these ideas help you and your family too. You can also find lots more activity ideas online, so keep trying new things and discover what you enjoy doing together. If you are doing an activity as a family, there is no wrong choice.

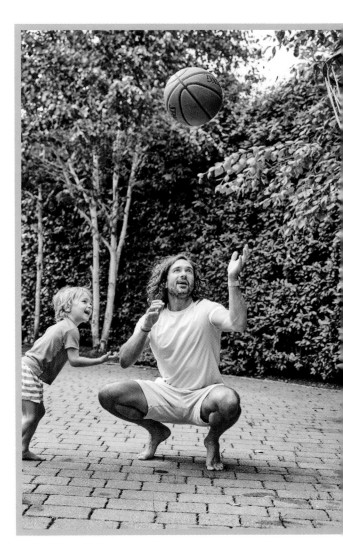

15 MINUTE WIN ←

Next time you feel you and the kids need it, if they are full of energy or you are feeling overwhelmed, give yourself 15 minutes of nature. This could be as simple as walking around the block, playing tag in the garden or making your way to the nearest park, forest or beach. There really is nothing better than fresh air and nature to clear the mind, and when you combine movement with nature, you have the perfect combination.

WALKING, DANCING, MOVING

Exercise doesn't need to be in a gym, and it doesn't need to be intense or serious or daunting. It can be fun, joyful, slow, playful, unplanned, unscheduled and free flowing. It should feel good! Gardening is exercise, playing hide-and-seek in the house with the kids is exercise, dancing to Taylor Swift in your bedroom is exercise (guilty as charged, Your Honour). All movement is good for you. The key to a healthy life is…

JUST KEEP MOVING!

GET INVENTIVE

If you find exercise boring or dull and struggle to commit, then it is time to think of other ways to bring healthy movement into your life. There is no excuse to not do anything because there is always some form of exercise you can enjoy. It can be really simple, the most important thing is to just keep moving!

To start, you can incorporate easy, focused movement into every aspect of your life. You don't need dedicated time. For example, when you are next in an online meeting (video off if you prefer), why don't you do some stretching or mobility exercises at the same time (see pages 198–209).

15 MINUTE WIN

Put this book down, stick on one of your favourite songs and give yourself a couple of minutes to just let loose. It might sound cringey – but trust me, it's so much fun and you will feel great afterwards. What is more therapeutic than dancing? It's a moment to let your hair down and move your body in whatever way makes you feel good. I promise you will come away smiling.

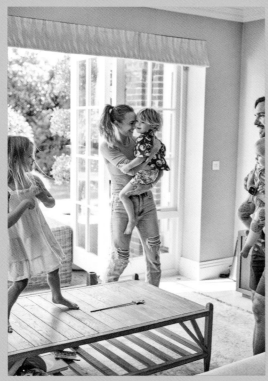

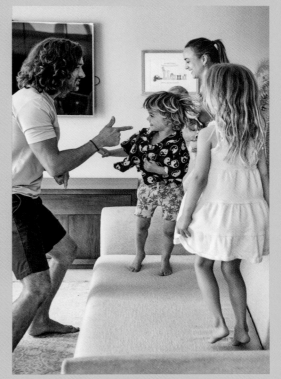

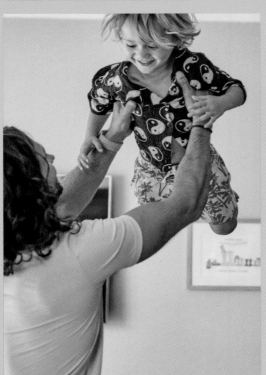

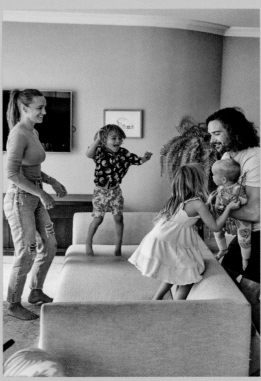

IDEAS FOR SMALL DAILY WINS

Set yourself up for success – the more you think about the small decisions you are making, the better. Take the opportunity to make tiny changes in your day-to-day life which will quickly and easily help you feel good and make your health and happiness a priority. Here are a selection of simple 15-minutes wins to help get you started.

MEALS (SEE PAGES 10-155)

1. Try making a new recipe
2. Stock up on different types of Tupperware
3. Add a new fruit and a new vegetable to the food shop
4. Ditch buying sweets and crisps as part of your weekly shop
5. Pack healthy snacks for you to eat on to go
6. Plan your food for the whole week

MOVEMENT (SEE PAGE 156)

1. Take a moment to stretch during your next online meeting (with camera off if you prefer!)
2. When you are chatting on the phone, get up and walk!
3. When you can, take the stairs
4. Sit up straight if you are slouching and think about your posture when standing
5. Walk the long way home from the station
6. Plan your exercise routines for the week

SLEEP (SEE PAGE 214)

1. Go to bed earlier
2. Invest in an eye mask
3. Buy an alarm clock
4. Disable the snooze button
5. Read a book before bed
6. Leave your phone downstairs
7. Talk to your partner about any worries
8. Tidy your bedroom

YOUR MIND (SEE PAGE 222)

1. Make your bed as soon as you get up
2. Drink a glass of water
3. Eat a healthy breakfast
4. Do something creative
5. Give yourself plenty of time to get to work, so that you don't need to rush
6. Call a friend or a loved one
7. Make time to reflect on your day
8. Perform a random act of kindness
9. Write down one positive thing about yourself or one thing that you are grateful for
10. Step away from your phone
11. Declutter or tidy your space
12. Spend time in nature
13. Send a heartfelt message to a loved one
14. Try a guided meditation
15. Listen to motivational music
16. Subscribe to a new podcast
17. Take a cold shower
18. Make mini icebergs (see page 236)

7. Schedule some downtime – whether alone, with your partner, or with your children
8. Block out all of your lunch breaks in your calendar and stick to it
9. Take yourself out on a date and do something that you love to do
10. Plan a small surprise for your partner
11. Plan a family activity for the weekend
12. Write a list of your priorities for the future

THE NIGHT BEFORE

1. Make your lunch – and breakfast too, if you need to eat on the go
2. Decide what to wear the next day and lay out your clothes
3. Leave the essentials by the door (keys, wallet, headphones)
4. Plan tomorrow night's dinner, and go to the shops on the way home tonight and buy the missing ingredients
5. There's only so much you can do in advance. For everything else, make yourself a to-do list so you can clear your mind of tasks

LIFESTYLE (SEE PAGE 238)

1. Check one easy thing off your to-do list
2. Now tackle your hardest task
3. Identify the things in your work or life that you can delegate
4. Turn off non-essential notifications
5. Make time for a hobby or passion project
6. Eat lunch away from your work desk

WHAT ONE THING COULD YOU DO RIGHT NOW THAT WOULD MAKE A POSITIVE DIFFERENCE TO YOUR DAY?

INDEX

INDEX

ACKNOWLEDGEMENTS

It has been an absolute pleasure creating this book with HarperCollins. I've had so much fun. I have been so lucky to get to work with David Loftus and Saskia Sidey for the first time, who are both fantastic to work with and so talented. The recipes, food styling, photography and design in this book are beautiful, so thank you to everyone involved.

Thank you, Lisa Milton and Louise McKeever, for driving the whole team and myself forward to really create the best work. I love how much you care about making the highest quality books. You never rush anything and always work so hard to push the standard up. I'm really proud of this book and can't wait to share it with others.

Thank you, Bev James, for being so supportive with my publishing career for all these years. Eleven books together now and we are still going strong.

Shout out to my wonderful wife and kids for being the reason I'm smiling in every photo. You are the happiness I've always searched for, and I love that we are on this journey through life together.

Keep moving forward.

Love,

Joe

ABOUT JOE WICKS

Known to multiple millions of fans as The Body Coach, Joe Wicks MBE is the author of 10 *Sunday Times* bestselling cookbooks and the founder of Lean in 15 and The Body Coach app. He also writes *The Burpee Bears* series for children.

Joe's passion for health and fitness led to him pursuing a degree in Sports Science before becoming a personal trainer. In March 2020, he delivered online PE lessons to over 100 million students and parents globally during the coronavirus pandemic and later gained a Guinness World Record for the largest YouTube livestream audience. In 2022, he was awarded an MBE.

Take your journey to the next level with The Body Coach App

Scan the QR code to get your exclusive £20 discount on the app.

£69.99 ~~£89.99~~ per year

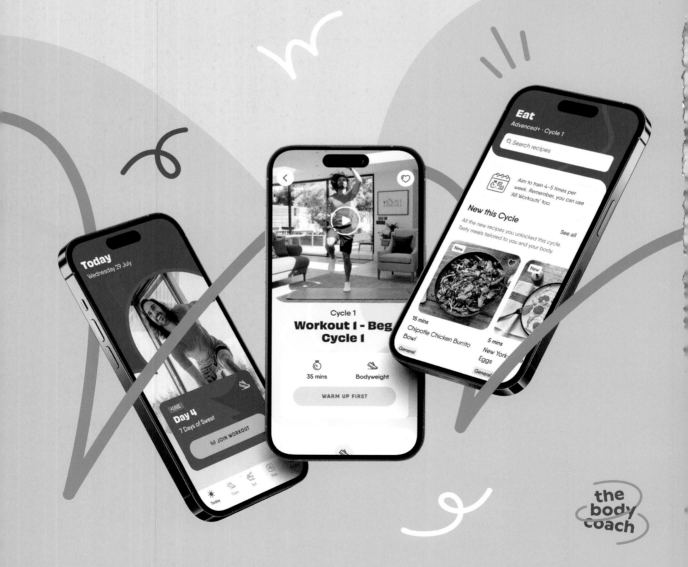